ALSO BY JERILYN ROSS

Triumph Over Fear

one less thing to
WORRY ABOUT

JERILYN ROSS, M.A.
with ROBIN CANTOR-COOKE

one less thing to WORRY ABOUT

UNCOMMON WISDOM FOR COPING WITH COMMON ANXIETIES

BALLANTINE BOOKS NEW YORK

One Less Thing to Worry About is a work of nonfiction. Some names and identifying details have been changed.

As of press time, the URLs displayed in this book link or refer to existing websites on the Internet. Random House, Inc., is not responsible for, and should not be deemed to endorse or recommend, any website other than its own or any content available on the Internet (including without limitation at any website, blog page, information page), or elsewhere, that is not created by Random House. The authors, similarly, cannot be responsible for third-party material.

Published in the United States by Ballantine Books, an imprint of The Random House Publishing Group, a division of Random House, Inc., New York.

BALLANTINE and colophon are registered trademarks of Random House, Inc.

The adapted sleep diary on page 98 is used with the permission of the National Sleep Foundation. For further information, please visit http://www.sleeepfoundation.org.

LIBRARY OF CONGRESS CATALOGING-IN-PUBLICATION DATA

Ross, Jerilyn.

One less thing to worry about: uncommon wisdom for coping with common anxieties / Jerilyn Ross with Robin Cantor-Cooke.

p. cm.

Includes bibliographical references and index.

ISBN 978-0-345-50306-0

1. Anxiety in women—Popular works. 2. Anxiety—Popular works. 3. Self-help techniques. I. Cantor-Cooke, Robin. II. Title.

BF575.A6R666 2009

152.4'6082—dc22 2009005575

Printed in the United States of America on acid-free paper

www.ballantinebooks.com

9 8 7 6 5 4 3 2 1

FIRST EDITION

Book design by Casey Hampton

To Ronnie
For keeping the promise

CONTENTS

AUTHOR'S NOTE

Writing this book is an act of advocacy by which I hope to provide women with strategies for managing everyday anxiety, bulletins on the latest anxiety research from top scientists, and my thoughts on what it all means. Some of my comments are grounded in science; others are born of my experiences as a therapist, patient advocate, and person who overcame a height phobia; and still others originate in the stories of my own patients and those of my colleagues, as well as my family members and friends.

To preserve the privacy and dignity of the people who have lived these stories, I have disguised their identities by altering some, but not all, characteristics of their lives: a middle-aged patient with a law practice might not get any younger in these pages but may be found practicing medicine instead; a friend with three children may be portrayed here as having either two or four. In some instances, I have merged aspects of several cases into one, creating a patient whose speech reflects experiences common to many women and whose story is a composite intended to convey the variety and texture of these women's lives without making them recognizable.

There is one exception: my friend Merle, whose fear of snakes you will read about in Chapter 6. When I asked her if she would prefer to be provided a pseudonym, she replied that she was perfectly comfortable being called by her actual name. For this I thank her, as I do the many other good and courageous women whose candor, fortitude, and humor enliven this book.

introduction

IN DEFENSE OF ANXIETY

For nearly thirty years I have worked with patients, medical doctors, researchers, psychologists, social workers, legislators, journalists, and media figures to raise awareness of and educate people about the causes, impact, and treatment of anxiety disorders. I have also worked to help people understand the difference between the normal anxiety, stress, and tension we all feel from time to time and the chronic, intense, irrational anxiety experienced by people suffering from an anxiety disorder.

And I'm the right person for the job: when I was in my early twenties, I was stricken with an inexplicable and paralyzing fear of heights while dancing on a mountaintop veranda high above the glistening lights of Salzburg in Austria. Little did I know that this relatively common but life-altering event would inspire my life's work. Triumphing over that irrational yet real and crippling fear, which dictated where I could live, which friends I could visit, and whom I could work for (I was living in Manhattan and unable to go above the tenth floor), marked the beginning of my professional relationship with anxiety.

When I set about writing my first book, *Triumph Over Fear,* very little had been published about anxiety disorders, so my goal was to create a resource that would tell people what to expect when they weren't anticipating a panic attack but inexplicably found themselves having one anyway. That book explored the outward manifestations and inner experience of anxiety disorders, focusing on panic disorder, phobias, obsessive-compulsive disorder (OCD), post-traumatic stress disorder (PTSD), and generalized anxiety disorder (GAD) and featured a step-by-step program to help people cope with these disorders and offer hope that the day might come when irrational, inexplicable anxiety no longer ruled their lives.

Since then, research into the causes and diagnosis of anxiety disorders, vast strides in their treatment, and programs to educate both health professionals and the public about them have brought these medical conditions out into the light of day, where we can get a good look at them. People have become more willing to talk about anxiety disorders and reach out for help. Famous athletes and entertainers routinely go on television and talk about their struggles with panic disorder and social phobia; fifteen years ago, this would have been unthinkable. Even the armed forces are more forthcoming: as I write this, a breaking story in *The New York Times* has reported a substantial increase in the number of servicemen and -women diagnosed with PTSD—nearly forty thousand cases since 2003. In a laudable display of candor, Pentagon officials said that these cases represent only those tracked by the military and estimate that many more of their people suffer from the disorder, citing embarrassment or fear of career damage as a reason for why more of them don't seek treatment. The officials said they were encouraging service members to seek help, even if they preferred to work with private therapists and not report the problem to the military.[1] This is all to the good: anxiety disorders are medical illnesses, not signs of weakness or character flaws, as people used to believe.

Nor do anxiety disorders develop from ordinary, everyday

anxiety, as people also once believed. You are not going to develop a height phobia, for example, because you feel dizzy and get butterflies in your stomach when you gaze down from the fortieth-floor balcony at your in-laws' apartment; nor will you develop obsessive-compulsive disorder because, as a nurse, you make a point of washing your hands frequently throughout the day. Anxiety disorders are not inevitable outgrowths of everyday anxiety any more than measles is the outgrowth of a heat rash: some of the symptoms may be similar, but their underlying causes are different. Likewise, the fact that you manifest some behaviors associated with an anxiety disorder does not mean that you have one, nor that you will develop one. What it may mean is that you are experiencing enough anxiety to adversely affect some of your thoughts and behaviors, which in turn may be making you less comfortable in your skin than you would like to be. If this is the case, you are wise to address your anxiety, however accustomed you may have become to living with it.

The science of anxiety and anxiety disorders is still relatively new. Even as I write about the latest research, scrupulously checking references, some of what I cite is being challenged, debated, and, in some cases, refuted in a laboratory, at a medical conference, or in a professional journal somewhere in the world. This is both the glory and the challenge of writing about a subject that is so vast, complex, and often controversial yet has implications that affect us so profoundly. Add to this the fact that, although we are making progress, there is still a dearth of information about the mechanism of anxiety in women—even though, when it comes to having anxiety disorders, we outnumber men two to one.

What we do know for sure is that anxiety can be our best friend or our worst foe. It can keep us out of trouble or land us knee-deep in it. It can motivate us to perform at peak level or leave us paralyzed with fear. Sometimes it's predictable; sometimes it pops up when we least expect it to. And though we all have different and evolving relationships with our anxiety, what we also have in common as part of a living, breathing species is that anxiety is part of our lives.

So, together, let us try to understand it, test it, challenge it, and accept it as just that: a necessary if sometimes perplexing part of life. Just as surviving a minor infection can protect you from developing a serious, disabling illness, so can learning to manage everyday anxieties protect you from developing anxiety-related problems and, in some cases, medical illnesses. The key is to understand that anxiety is not a noxious emotional state but rather a normal, healthy response to myriad stressors exerting themselves upon us all the time, every day. Just as it is unrealistic to imagine a life without stress, so it is unrealistic to imagine a life without anxiety. For a woman to try to banish it from her existence would be tantamount to exiling herself from the human condition.

part one

ANXIETY: A GIRL'S BEST FRIEND—OR FOE?

one

ANXIETY'S NEW NORMAL

The idea for this book came to me in a gallbladder—my husband's gallbladder, actually.

I was waiting for Ronnie to come out of surgery to remove a whopper of a gallstone that had shown up during a routine physical. The doctor had said we could leave it alone and maybe nothing would ever happen, or he could operate and take out the gallbladder and Ronnie wouldn't have to worry about needing emergency surgery someday. Now, when I go to the doctor, I ask ten million questions; the more I know, the less anxious I feel. But my husband is a practical man. He needs only enough information to make a rational decision. "Why take a chance?" he asked. "It's a simple procedure; why would I want to be traveling through Europe and suddenly find myself in a foreign hospital in agony? Let's do it. When can we schedule the surgery?"

Which is how I came to be sitting in a room with about a dozen other people, all waiting to either go in for surgery themselves or hear about how their loved ones had weathered their procedures. I was mildly anxious but not overly so; I knew Ronnie's surgery wasn't risky because I had pelted the doctor with questions: "Does he need his gallbladder for anything?" (No.) "What does laparoscopic surgery entail?" (Several small incisions; very simple, very routine.) "How long will the surgery last?" (An hour; hour and a half at most.)

I like information when I'm anxious; it comforts me. It provides a framework on which I can layer facts and opinions and second opinions that enable me to make good decisions. As Ronnie's surgery approached, I learned everything I could about gallstones, gallbladders, and anything else the surgeon happened to mention. I'm pretty familiar with my anxiety (after thirty years as an anxiety professional, that's no surprise), and I know that when I'm anxious, information is my friend: not only does it enable me to understand what's going on, but it also helps me ensure that my loved ones are getting the best possible care.

I had carried with me into the waiting room a satchel containing a bundle of magazines and newspapers, a PDA full of emails that I needed to answer, a novel, a container of almonds, a bottle of orange juice, and a stack of journal articles I had to read for work. I had brought all this stuff because I didn't think I'd be able to sit and concentrate on any one thing, and I was right. I opened the novel, stared at the same sentence for five minutes, and put it back; pulled out *Newsweek* and then *The New Yorker,* read a few paragraphs, put them back; took a sip of juice; prodded my PDA, glanced at an email, put back the PDA; grabbed *The New York Times,* looked at the headlines, opened it, closed it, and thrust it back into the satchel. Losing myself in reading wasn't going to work; I wanted to be occupied but present, somewhat distracted but available to see the surgeon the moment he entered the waiting room.

That's another thing: I'd chosen a chair that faced the elevators so I could see whoever was coming off. From where I was sitting, not only would I see the surgeon as soon as the doors opened; I'd be able to study his expression so by the time he reached me, I would be prepared for whatever he had to say. If he looked happy, I could leap from the chair with joy; if he looked grim, I could brace myself for bad news. I could imagine either outcome, but I simply could not imagine sitting with my back to the elevators because I knew when those doors opened and the surgeon strode out, I needed to be the first one to see him.

The doors slid open; no sign of the surgeon. I checked my watch and saw that the hour was up. What was taking so long? Was everything okay? I approached the perky woman behind the check-in counter.

"Gee, it's taking longer than I thought," I said.

"The doctor reserved the operating room for two hours. Sometimes things go slower, or they may have started late." She smiled brightly.

I returned to my seat. They'd said it could take ninety minutes and only an hour had passed, so there was no reason to worry. None at all. In my rational mind, I knew that everything was probably fine, that surgery is a complex undertaking and there was no reason to think that everything would be finished after only an hour. Even so, something could go terribly wrong: an unexpected growth, a problem with the anesthesia, a hemorrhage . . .

I looked around the room. A middle-aged man sat near me reading *The Washington Post,* eyes flicking across the neatly folded panel of newsprint. Across the room a woman sat several chairs away from a boy of about fifteen, whom I took to be her son; because of his pronounced limp and wincing when they came in, I figured he was the patient. He sprawled in his chair, legs outstretched, eyes and thumbs darting about a handheld gaming system. His hair was unkempt, and his jeans looked as if they had not been washed for a month. Woman and boy neither looked at nor acknowledged the other; had I not seen them arrive, I would not have known they were together. It was obvious that they were both dealing with their anxiety in the way that adolescents and parents do when, for instance, they are watching a movie and are ambushed by a sex scene: suddenly there's an elephant in the room and everyone slouches down in his or her seat and stares straight ahead until the agony abates. This kid seemed oblivious to where he was and why he was there until a uniformed nurse approached him and he jumped up, grimacing. His mother, who had seemed equally oblivious, also leapt to her feet and stood beside him protectively.

There was a woman who had been talking nonstop on her cell phone since she entered the room; another sat silently twisting the rings on her fingers. A man in work boots pulled a pamphlet from a display, sat down, read it, returned it to the rack, then took another and repeated the cycle all over again. It was fascinating to realize that we were all in this room, waiting and anxious, yet no two people were exhibiting the same behaviors.

My gaze drifted back to the man with the newspaper. He was well dressed and seemed no more troubled than if he were waiting for a train. He held the paper the way people do on a crowded subway, folded in half lengthwise and then crosswise so it formed a neat rectangle of newsprint. I watched as he started to read a story, smoothing the paper with his hand and unfolding and refolding the pages as he read each column. Then, when he finished a story, he unfolded the paper, opened it to the next page, refolded it into a rectangle, and began reading again. His movements were deliberate and economical, and I watched him repeat them as he made his way through the news section and then on through Metro and Business.

I was amazed. How can he sit there reading? I wondered. He must be waiting to hear about someone important to him; why is he so detached? How can he concentrate? Doesn't he care? If he's so unconcerned, why is he even here?

My reverie ended as a woman in a white jacket with a stethoscope walked toward him. He looked up, set the newspaper down, and stood, smoothing his trouser legs. I was sitting there thinking, Hurry up! Hurry up and get over there! A few seconds later I heard her say, "She's fine, everything looks benign," and the man's eyes were trained on her face and he was nodding his head rapidly and saying "Thank you, thank you, Doctor" and vigorously shaking her hand. Then she walked away and the man sat back down, stared into space for about half a minute, picked up the newspaper, and resumed reading.

I thought, Thank you? That's it? Just *thank you*? How can he be so blasé? Does he not have feelings? Does he not love his wife? Is he having an affair and disappointed that his wife will be hanging around longer than he thought? Or does he love his wife so much that he can't allow himself to think that something bad could happen to her? Does he keep himself together by being stoic, or did he have two martinis when he woke up this morning? Is it his personality? His upbringing? His genetics? Is he religious and convinced that God wouldn't let something bad happen to a person as good as his wife? Why isn't he anxious? Why isn't he acting more normal?

I checked my watch: an hour and forty-seven minutes had passed. Nothing to worry about, but . . . My mind started wandering to the stories I'd heard about somebody's uncle who went in for gallbladder surgery but when they opened him up they found something else; and another man who got an infection in the hospital and ended up dying from that. My rational mind knew that the chances of this happening to Ronnie were remote, but you never know. I started planning the eulogy.

I had gotten to the part where I was saying what a wonderful guy Ronnie was, how grateful I was to have found him relatively late in life, how he had raised three wonderful kids, and how I blamed myself because maybe if I had taken him to the doctor a little earlier, fatal complications would not have set in, when a small voice inside me piped up: Your husband is having a gallstone removed and you're planning the eulogy. You think that's normal?

Sure, it was normal—*for me.*

I was working on how to break the news to the children when all of a sudden the surgeon emerged from the elevator and I was on my feet in an instant and then he was right in front of me saying "Everything's okay, it went just fine." And I was thinking, I need more words, more than just "okay" and "fine." And he went to shake my hand and I said, "No, I've got to hug you," and I put my arms around him and, next thing you know, I was shaking and crying and bombarding him with questions: "He's all right? No problems with the anesthesia? You didn't find anything else? He's still unconscious? When can I see him?" And I kept shaking and the doctor kept saying, "He's really okay, he's really okay," and he was looking at me as if I were a little crazy for crying so much over a gallbladder, for God's sake, and in the midst of all the relief and tears and gratitude I was thinking, This is strange: I spend so much time talking to patients, colleagues, and reporters about what's normal and what's not normal, and here I am, acting in a way that may seem overemotional or ridiculous to others and yet that's completely normal for me when I'm worried about someone I love.

That's when the idea for this book was born, because in that moment I realized that when it comes to everyday anxiety, there is no such thing as normal; rather, there is a broad spectrum of normal, within which most of us can be found. I occupy a slot on the spectrum where anxiety manifests as an eruption of raw emotion, and I know this is normal for me. Each of us manifests and responds differently to anxiety because *each of us has a different relationship with our anxiety,* just as each of us has a different relationship with our mothers, our fathers, our children, and everyone else in our lives. What's important is not learning the "right" way to respond to anxiety but learning how *you* relate to it and whether or not the relationship is working.

The mother and son who seemed so oblivious in the waiting room, the woman who talked incessantly on her cell phone, the man reading the pamphlets, the woman twisting her rings: all of them had different relationships with their anxiety and were doing something within the context of that relationship to manage their anxious feelings. They didn't necessarily realize they were doing it, but each of them was manifesting behaviors that were specifically chosen, however unconsciously, to manage their anxiety and keep it from getting the better of them.

It became clear to me that the middle-aged fellow was not engrossed in the newspaper in spite of his anxiety but because of it: I had no proof, of course, but it now seemed obvious that his systematic reading, folding, and smoothing of the newspaper were components of a ritual that helped him control the anxiety he was probably feeling. His repeated thanks to the doctor and energetic shaking of her hand were evidence of the intensity with which he received the news of the patient's well-being. The fact that he was able to sit there reading the newspaper—or appearing to read it, at any rate—was not evidence of a lack of empathy but rather a demonstration of how he related to his anxiety: as a force that could be controlled, if not conquered, by executing a series of small and manageable actions. His deliberate, measured movements were for him what my questioning the doctor and planning the eulogy were for me: a coping mechanism uniquely suited to his personality and situation and designed to keep his anxiety under control.

Each of us has a variety of coping mechanisms, patterns of behaviors that get us through the anxiety-provoking situations that life inevitably nudges our way. You may be someone who deals with anxiety by avoiding thoughts and situations that remind you of it, or you may ruminate about your anxiety in an attempt to think it into submission. Whether you avoid your anxiety or think about it will depend on how you perceive yourself in relation to the anxiety. Is it so powerful that your only way of coping is to avoid it? Or do you see yourself as playing a role in managing it? In either case, the important question is whether or not the relationship is working for you. That question may not be easy to answer.

CORINNA: "IF THE CANCER COMES BACK, IT COMES BACK. I'M NOT GOING TO WASTE PRECIOUS TIME RUNNING TO DOCTORS"

I have a neighbor whom I'll call Corinna. Four years ago, when she was in her mid-fifties, she found an irregularly shaped mole on her thigh and, after much prodding from her husband, agreed to see a dermatologist. It turned out to be cancerous and was surgically removed. She did not say much about it at the time other than that they seemed to have caught the disease early and that her doctor was pleased.

I saw Corinna recently, told her I was writing a book about women and anxiety, and said I was interested in hearing about how she dealt with her health concerns and the anxiety she felt before her dermatologist appointments.

"I haven't been back to the dermatologist," she said.

It was as if she had hit me over the head with a sledgehammer.

"Didn't you have skin cancer a while back?"

"Yes, a few years ago."

"What kind did you have?"

"You know, I'm not really sure."

"Was it basal cell or squamous cell? Or melanoma?"

"I think it was melanoma."

I was speechless. Melanoma is the most serious form of skin cancer because it can spread more quickly to other parts of the body than either basal or squamous cell carcinomas. Corinna is an accomplished, highly educated woman. Why would someone so intelligent stick her head in the sand like this?

"Corinna, melanoma is serious. How can you have had a melanoma and not follow up with your dermatologist?"

"If I see something new, I'll go to the doctor and he'll take it off, like he did last time."

"But you can't always see when a melanoma has spread. What if you don't catch it in time? What if it's somewhere where you can't see it and by the time you do catch it it's too late?"

"If it comes back, it comes back. I caught it last time, and I'll catch it again. I'm not going to waste precious time running to doctors so they can cut off little pieces of me until there's nothing left. I look fine and I feel fine. There's nothing I can do about this except stay out of the sun, and I do that. Why shouldn't I enjoy my life as much as I can?"

I looked at Corinna. This is a woman with a lot of medical problems: high blood pressure, adult-onset diabetes, and an arthritic hip that sometimes makes it difficult for her to walk. Yet every time I talk to her, she has just returned from a trip to Asia or a bird-watching expedition to Central America. I saw her once when she was released from the hospital after a bout of double pneumonia. She and her husband had travel plans yet again, and she said, "I'm not missing this trip—if I die, I die." And she went, and she didn't die, and now she was saying pretty much the same thing about her skin cancer: I'm going to enjoy my life. We all die eventually, and when my time is up, it's up.

Can I relate to Corinna's fatalistic, *que será, será* philosophy? No, I cannot: it's completely foreign to me. When something is ailing me or someone I love, I seek out every iota of information so I can learn about it, weigh the options, make sensible decisions, and feel as if I'm participating in life rather than allowing life to happen to me.

But I also think that there are a lot of people like Corinna. Corinna claims she is not anxious about her skin cancer or her other medical problems; she neither complains nor asks her friends to cater to her. In fact, many people admire Corinna's stoicism and comment on what they perceive as her honesty and courage. But I am a bit more cynical: the way I see it, either she is anxious and denying the feelings, or she really isn't anxious and would be better off if she were.

Better off with more anxiety? Actually, yes: there are times when we need anxiety to motivate us to protect and take better care of ourselves (or others, as the case may be). It's that twinge of anxiety that tells you that it's time for your medical follow-up exam or that it would be wise to avoid deserted sections of the parking garage even if it means having to wait for a spot on the first floor, where there's an attendant. It's anxiety that tells you perhaps you should call and make sure an adult will be home before you send your fourteen-year-old daughter off to a sleepover at a friend's house. While it is true that many of us have too much anxiety, some of us don't have enough for our own good, which is why I neither embrace nor entirely trust Corinna's fatalistic attitude. Despite her protestations to the contrary, I do not believe that Corinna was or is ready for her life to end: anyone who loves to travel as much as she does is, in my opinion, still hungry for new experiences and engaged in life. What I do believe is that Corinna's seeming lack of anxiety about her melanoma could have life-and-death consequences.

The point, of course, is not whether or not I embrace Corinna's approach to her medical care but whether or not it is working for her. Every woman must decide how proactive she wants to be when it comes to her medical care, and no woman can do that until she understands that her relationship with her anxiety affects the way she makes such decisions. That's why I believe that every woman owes it to herself to examine this relationship and determine whether or not her anxiety (or in Corinna's case, her seeming lack of it) is working for her and preserving her well-being or working against her and making her vulnerable to harm.

Well, you may be thinking, not everyone has serious health concerns like this Corinna person. Is it really that important to examine the alleged relationship I have with my anxiety? Why not just let it work itself out?

In fact, a good deal of the anxiety we experience does work itself out—such as the anxiety you might feel while waiting to learn if you got a promotion or when your sixteen-year-old takes the car out alone for the first time. That kind of anxiety tends to dissipate once the situation causing it is over. But some anxiety doesn't dissipate sufficiently to allow us to relax and recover from its effects. Long-term, unrelieved anxiety can settle over our lives like a fog, obscuring our perceptions and convincing us that danger is lurking everywhere, biding its time before pouncing and wreaking havoc on our lives.

And who can blame us? Who hasn't been wracked with revulsion at the high-definition horror broadcast into our homes? Men and women strap explosives to their bodies, blow themselves and scores of other people to pieces, and we are soon bombarded with images of destruction and anguish. It seems as if every morning brings headlines of some fresh new atrocity from the other side of the world or the other end of town.

It's not that danger never threatened us before; it's just that we weren't so relentlessly aware of it. We program our computers to alert us to breaking news stories; our cell phones and PDAs jiggle and chirp and inform us of events while they are still happening; and television shows are interrupted by jarring bulletins on everything from government scandals to school shootings to scattered hailstorms that may or may not come our way.

Don't misunderstand me: I think it's great to be able to get information swiftly and easily when you want and need it. But more and more, we're being inundated with information we neither want nor need, which, because it is suddenly *there,* acquires an aura of urgency that demands a response.

We're paying a high price for all this knowledge, and I don't mean just our Internet bills: we are paying with our peace of mind. We are so plugged in to things that are happening here, there, and everywhere that we are losing the capacity, not to mention the will, to seek out solitude, separate from the hubbub, and calm ourselves. Sure, we can turn off our phones, PDAs, and laptops, but what if something happens? What if someone needs us? What if we're not available at the very moment someone—anyone—calls?

The relentless onslaught of stimuli makes us feel vital, alive, *happening.* But what's really happening is that we are living in a state of perpetual hyperawareness, primed to pick up signals from the minimachines in our pockets, ears, and purses. The result is that we are constantly poised to respond and react, to fight or flee, jittery and anxious all the time.

This is anxiety's new normal. For example, we now consider it normal to fret if we leave the house without a cell phone, even if we aren't expecting a call. It wasn't that long ago that parents went out to dinner and a movie utterly phoneless, leaving the babysitter with the name of the restaurant and movie they would be attending and figuring the sitter could locate them by calling and asking for the manager in case of an emergency. Now it's hard to imagine going out for the evening and leaving your cell phone behind along with the kids. Why? Are our children really in greater danger at home with a sitter now than they were twenty years ago? Is it really necessary for the sitter to be able to reach us in twenty seconds rather than two minutes?

I don't think so. Going out for dinner and a movie may pose a greater danger to your budget now than it used to, but it's certainly no more dangerous for the kids at home. What has changed is that it's now considered perfectly normal to have a telephone with you at all times, even to have it affixed to your ear like a gleaming growth. (It is also, alas, considered normal to stride through airports and other public places speaking aloud to someone miles away and exposing everyone in general to your private business, whether they want to hear it or not.)

Now, before I utter another word critical of cell-phone syndrome, let me say this: I love my cell phone. It has brought a level of comfort and security and tranquillity into my life that I would be loath to relinquish. It has also granted me and millions of others relief in a host of anxiety-provoking situations. If I'm stuck in traffic and late for a meeting, for instance, I no longer have to get even more worked up trying to decide whether to take the time to find a pay phone and a quarter so I can call in to the office or to just grit my teeth and stay the course; now I just whip out my phone and let them know I'm on my way. We have the almost unimaginable potential to be hooked in to everyone we know and care about and anything we might want to know or care about in little more than the time it takes to think of it—and all because of the dazzling speed and efficiency of these machines, which are small and light enough to carry with us all the time. But because it is now normal to always have a phone with us, we have developed a dependency on it and the lightning-fast communication it provides, so much that we begin to feel insecure without it. The potential to connect, in other words, can create a false need to feel connected. This artificial need to be constantly connected, hooked in, and reachable exemplifies anxiety's new normal, and it's doing us some harm along with the good.

It's doing women even less good than it's doing men, as women seem inclined to be more anxious than men in the first place: we're the ones who wake up first when a baby is crying or a child is standing silently alongside the bed in the middle of the night. We're also the ones who tend to worry about whether the people around us are hungry or thirsty or need a nap or a sweater or something for a headache. Let's also not forget that many women are also breadwinners and work two or more jobs, one of which, if they have a family, offers no salary, sick days, or opportunity for advancement. As hard as men work at their jobs, women are far more likely to be worrying about whether there's enough milk in the fridge, socks in the drawer, and detergent in the laundry room and to be keeping track of the family's social engagements, doctor's appointments, and parent-teacher conferences, not to mention arranging play dates, vacations, and veggie platters long after we've gotten home from our other jobs. And make no mistake: our other jobs aren't hobbies. Whether we are on salary or paid by the hour, we are working outside the home as well as within it because, for many families, the rent wouldn't get paid if we didn't.

So women are experiencing more and more anxiety as they juggle the stresses of working a job, managing a household, living in a newly violent world, and having everything brought to their attention 24/7. What else is new?

What's new is the knowledge that anxiety can make you more than jittery; it can also make you sick. We used to think that anxious women had nothing to fear but fear itself, but recent research indicates that chronic, excessive anxiety may be a catalyst for a host of serious medical problems, including cardiovascular disease; mood disorders, including bipolar disorder and depression; eating disorders; drug abuse; asthma; irritable bowel syndrome; and alcoholism. (For more on anxiety and co-occurring medical conditions, see Chapter 8.)

The connection between anxiety and depression is especially significant. We know that women are twice as likely as men to be anxious, with millions of women suffering depression along with anxiety. For years we believed that this meant that, as with anxiety, women were twice as likely as men to become depressed.

But new research suggests otherwise: in 2001, Gordon Parker, M.D., Ph.D., an Australian psychiatrist and professor, reanalyzed the results of a North American study and found that *women's greater vulnerability to depression is likely a result of their predisposition to anxiety.* Parker went back to the study of eight thousand women and took another look at the data, which led him to conclude that *the odds of a woman experiencing depression are directly related to whether or not she experienced anxiety earlier in life.* Not only that—Parker found that girls begin exceeding boys' incidence of anxiety and depression in early adolescence, a predominance that peaks between the ages of twenty-five and forty, suggesting that female sex hormones—notably estrogen—may play a significant role in triggering anxiety in women.[1]

The inference—and it's an important one—is that women may be more vulnerable to depression because their fluctuating hormones render them more vulnerable to anxiety. This may also explain why women seem to be especially vulnerable to anxiety during adolescence, pregnancy, postpartum, breast-feeding, and the menopausal transition. (For more about anxiety and the female life cycle, see Chapter 3.)

"I NEVER USED TO BE LIKE THIS"

Ever since my first book came out and I landed an appearance on *The Oprah Winfrey Show,* people have approached me in airports, restaurants, and shoe departments to tell me about their struggles with phobias and panic attacks and their relief at knowing that there was at least one other person who knew what they were going through.

But many of the people I meet now are talking about a different struggle, and more and more of them are women. They do not necessarily seem to be suffering from a disorder so much as beset by an unsettling, if not disabling, feeling of unease. They persist in their everyday activities; they go to work and run their households and tend their children. Still, they find themselves fretting about things that never used to bother them and making decisions that pander to their fears. An executive told me she had turned down a promotion because the new job required monthly trips to California and ever since September 11, 2001, she has been too anxious to fly; a graduate teaching assistant at a small liberal arts college said that, ever since the calamity at Virginia Tech, she no longer feels safe in her classroom; a sixty-year-old homemaker said she is thinking about going off her antidepressant medication even though it is helping her, because she is anxious about side effects she has been reading about (and has yet to experience). They say, "I never used to be like this. I used to be able to go places and do things without worrying about every little thing that might go wrong. But now I find myself looking at people differently and fretting about stuff I never used to think about. It's like I've become this other person I don't recognize. Am I normal? Is there something wrong with me? Do I need professional help?"

The short answer is, I don't know: a therapist cannot know if a woman's anxiety is normal or excessive without sitting down with her for at least one or two sessions and learning about her symptoms, the thoughts and feelings that accompany the symptoms, and myriad other factors that, when considered together, situate the constellation of her anxious feelings within the universe of her life.

But the long answer—and the more satisfying one, I believe—is that when it comes to anxiety, there is a broad spectrum of normal. At one end of the spectrum are women whose anxiety seldom gets in the way; at the other end are those whose anxiety feels like a constant, prickly companion. Occupying the middle of the spectrum are the rest of us, women whose anxiety unsettles them more than they would like it to and who want to know what they can do about it.

I want you to know that there *are* things you can and should do about anxiety—not only because I have spent nearly thirty years helping people overcome the disabling effects of anxiety disorders but because we are learning that everyday, ordinary anxiety is not as benign as we thought. We used to think that the disorders were the only harmful form of anxiety, but we were wrong: new research is showing that the nervousness, tension, and worry that many of us live with and joke about are far from funny. Scientists have found that anxiety disorders as well as depression and other mood disorders can actually change the structure of certain parts of the brain, leading to diminished capacity to think and reason clearly. Just as striking are findings that in laboratory animals, these structural changes appear to be reversible when they are treated with antidepressant and antiseizure medications.[2]

Even more astonishing are indications that psychotherapy can do the same thing. In an intriguing experiment, Canadian researchers recruited twelve women who qualified as having arachnophobia (an intense fear of spiders) and had them watch film excerpts featuring spiders in all their eight-legged glory, after which the women's brains were given magnetic resonance imaging (MRI) scans. The scans revealed significant activity in the region associated with fear. Over the next four weeks, the women participated in weekly cognitive-behavioral therapy (CBT) sessions during which they were progressively exposed to color pictures of spiders, films of live spiders, and actual spiders and, at the final session, asked to touch a tarantula—yes, you read that correctly—and what's more, they actually did it. After completing the therapy sessions, the women were again shown film excerpts of spiders and given MRIs, which showed a dramatic reduction of their brains' fear activity. This led the researchers to conclude that not only does CBT change the dysfunctional brain circuitry that triggers a phobia but that these changes are able to "functionally 'rewire' the brain."[3]

We have also known for some time about the connection between cortisol, a stress hormone, and the body's ability to fight disease. When a person is in a stressful situation, the adrenal glands produce cortisol (also known as hydrocortisone), which increases blood pressure and blood sugar levels, readying the body to combat a potential threat; at the same time, it also temporarily suppresses the body's immune function. As the immediate danger or stressful situation is relieved, the brain tells the adrenals to decrease the production of cortisol and other stress hormones, restoring the body's chemical balance. Research shows, however, that when stress continues for long periods unabated, the body is unable to regulate its stress hormone production effectively, inhibiting its immune response and leading to the continuing release of stress-relieving chemicals that promote inflammation, which may in turn lead to other medical problems. (For a detailed explanation of how the brain responds to stress, see Chapter 3.)

THE EMERGING PICTURE

We don't yet have all the puzzle pieces in place, but we do know that anxiety and stress are associated with medical illness and psychological dysfunction.

New research is also showing that women's anxiety manifests itself differently from men's and, as mentioned earlier, seems to vary across the life cycle, waxing and waning with shifts in hormone levels and the life-altering processes that tend to accompany them, such as menstruation, pregnancy, breast-feeding, and the menopausal transition. This emerging connection between anxiety and hormonal dynamics may explain why one healthy young woman develops obsessive-compulsive disorder during her pregnancy while another woman with a history of panic disorder ceases having panic attacks during hers. It may also explain why a woman who has lived for fifty years without anxiety problems may develop them as she begins to approach menopause. (For more about the chemical and biological roots of anxiety, see Chapter 3.)

Having said that, I also want to remind you that there are kinds of anxiety you need *not* be anxious about—that is, that some anxiety is not only not bad for us but is absolutely necessary for our well-being and survival. The anxious twinge that tells you not to lend money to your unreliable cousin could save you a bundle; the prickle of anxiety that tells you not to accept a ride home with that attractive but strange guy you just met may save your life. To set out to eradicate anxiety from your life would be as foolhardy as it would be unrealistic.

The goal, then, is not to fortify yourself against anxiety as if it were an enemy but rather to approach it as you might a beloved but difficult parent: terminating the relationship is out of the question, but figuring out how to get along better would profoundly improve an important aspect of your life. How can we do this? By understanding that anxiety isn't something that happens to us but something with which we are actively engaged, something with which we have a relationship. The way you relate to your anxiety—by avoiding it, placating it, facing it down, or responding to it in any number of different ways—determines the role you allow anxiety to play in your life. Do you defer to your anxiety as you might to a domineering husband, or do you placate it as you might a volatile lover? Do you avoid your anxiety as you might an irritating coworker? Or do you confront it, albeit shakily, as you once did that creep in fifth grade who made fun of what you had in your lunch box?

Learning to live with anxiety is like learning how to get along with the mothers, sisters, fathers, brothers, in-laws, friends, coworkers, supervisors, and assorted colorful and eccentric characters who make our lives worth living. It is a dynamic process, vibrant and changeable, steadfast in its unpredictability, pulsing with equal parts strife and exhilaration. It is, at the end of the day, a part of every woman's life. And the moment you understand that you have a living, breathing relationship with your anxiety—a relationship whose qualities and character are of your making—is the moment you free yourself from the tyranny of fear and assert your right to challenge, subdue, and even embrace it.

two

"AM I JUST A WORRIER, OR IS THERE SOMETHING WRONG WITH ME?"

If anxiety is a natural and inescapable part of every woman's life, how do you know whether and when to be concerned that the anxiety you feel is more than normal? How can you tell if the unease you experience around your newborn baby is natural for a first-time mother or a manifestation of a deeper, more pervasive problem? How do you know if your latest bout of insomnia is a symptom of stress at work or of a more complex condition? How do you know if your lifelong habit of washing your hands before and after every meal is good hygiene or a symptom of obsessive-compulsive disorder?

When I began treating phobias in the late 1970s, *The Washington Post* did a story on a patient of mine who had agoraphobia—an avoidance of places where one fears having a panic attack and being unable to get to safety—and who had been unable to leave her house for over thirty years (I wrote about her in *Triumph Over Fear*). As a result of the newspaper story, I began getting calls from reporters wanting to do stories on phobias, panic attacks, and anxiety in general. The press was fascinated by the subject. Many reporters prefaced their queries with the admission that they too suffered from an anxiety problem.

Over time I began to notice patterns in media coverage. As summer approached and folks got ready to go on vacation, there would be an increase in calls about fear of flying, driving over bridges, and driving through tunnels. Every year right before Thanksgiving and Christmas, reporters would call and ask for pointers about what people could do about holiday stress. I would always know when Friday the thirteenth was coming because my phone would start ringing on Thursday the twelfth with reporters asking about paraskavedekatriaphobia (fear of Friday the thirteenth—not to be confused with triskaidekaphobia, fear of the number thirteen, or the unnamed fear of not being able to pronounce either of them) and the origins and significance of the superstition surrounding that particular day. And when calamity strikes, as it did on 9/11, during the sniper attacks in Washington, D.C., and after the collapse of a bridge in Saint Paul, Minnesota, my phone starts ringing and email chirping with requests from radio, television, and print journalists who want their listeners, viewers, and readers to know how to cope with the anxiety these events inevitably cause. In fact, I was working on the outline for this book when I heard on the radio about the killings at Virginia Tech. Within moments, I began getting calls from journalists and didn't get back to the book for several hours.

As I look back, the other pattern that jumps out at me is that whether I was being interviewed by a magazine writer after a tragedy, a radio host about the latest treatments for anxiety disorders, or a television reporter during a show on bridge phobias, at some point the interviewer would ask some variation of the question "What is the difference between normal anxiety and an anxiety disorder?"

While my answers have evolved over the years, one thing remains constant: we all have anxiety and need it to function and survive, but when anxiety is persistent, excessive, and irrational and interferes with a person's day-to-day life, it is most likely an anxiety disorder.

Most of us would agree that a young mother's anxiety is probably normal when, for example, she's not sure she's holding her baby correctly when she burps him, whether his rash is a sign of a serious illness, or what to do when he won't stop crying. However, if the same young mother refuses to be alone with her child for fear of harming him, won't pick him up because she's afraid she might have germs on her hands and will contaminate him, or is afraid to call the pediatrician when her child is running a fever for fear of saying the wrong thing and making a fool of herself, she may indeed have an anxiety disorder.

Most of the time, the difference is obvious, especially to the person with the problem. The young mother who won't pick up her baby is aware that her behavior is irrational yet feels powerless to change it. She may go to great lengths to hide the seemingly senseless and often embarrassing behavior, making excuses for why she cannot pick up the baby after she's touched something she considers "germy"—complaining of back pain, for instance—and manipulating her husband, friends, and family members into doing it for her.

At times the person may try to justify the behavior to herself, even though she is aware that the anxiety doesn't make sense. For example, a young woman who refuses to be alone with her child for fear of harming her might think, I know there is no way in a million years I would or could ever harm my child, but there's no telling what might happen when that awful feeling comes over me—I just can't risk losing control. Yes, the feeling is terrifying, but as I tell my patients, although the feeling is frightening, it is not dangerous. People with anxiety disorders have scary thoughts, but they're just that—thoughts that have gone awry. They are not predictors of imminent actions. They are just thoughts; and thoughts alone, however scary, don't make people do things they don't want to do.

So if you have irrational, anxious thoughts about places, objects, or situations that pose no real threat of danger and that lead you to behave in ways that you perceive as irrational, you may have an anxiety disorder. We'll talk more about the specific symptoms of the different types of anxiety disorders later in this chapter, but for now, let's continue with getting a clearer picture of what is and what is not normal anxiety.

The fact that so many journalists continue to ask this question tells me that no matter how many times and in how many ways I and others try to answer it, either we haven't succeeded or all of us need constant reassurance that the anxiety symptoms we periodically experience are normal. We want to know we're okay. And once we know we're okay, we want to know how to calm our anxieties. Normal or not, anxiety feels bad and adversely affects our sense of well-being. In many cases, it also erodes our health.

Whereas we have language to describe the symptoms and manifestations of anxiety in general, we have no reliable diagnostic tools to measure the nature and severity of any one person's experience of it. There aren't any blood tests or X-rays that can tell me, for example, how the intensity of one person's panic attack compares to that of another, although we are moving in that direction. Researchers at Massachusetts General Hospital have found that the brains of people with post-traumatic stress disorder and those who suffer from a phobia manifest atypical activity in the areas that deal with fear, suggesting that such people experience apprehension more intensely than the rest of us.[1] And Jill M. Hooley, Ph.D., at Harvard has found scientific evidence of what a lot of us have known since we were kids: that the brain's anxiety mechanism starts cranking when people listen to an audiotape of a parent criticizing them.[2]

That said, one way to approach the issue is to ask yourself: "To what extent is anxiety interfering in my life?" Do you feel uncomfortable whenever you enter an elevator but stay on anyway, or did you quit your job when you learned your company was moving to a high-rise building? Do you make a point of washing your hands before eating and after taking the subway, or do you feel compelled to scrub them every time you touch a doorknob or shake hands with someone? Do you sometimes have trouble falling asleep after a rough day at work, or do you have chronic insomnia that leaves you perpetually exhausted no matter how your day goes?

You might also want to ask yourself whether or not you believe your anxiety is rational. Sure, it makes sense to be apprehensive about driving over an icy bridge at three in the morning in the midst of a hailstorm. But is it rational to drive half an hour out of your way, morning and evening, to avoid a bridge that, if you took it, would cut your commute in half? And no one would argue that chest pain, heart palpitations, and hyperventilation are signals that you should get yourself seen by a doctor right away. But something is awry when a healthy twenty-five-year-old woman with no family history of cardiovascular disease ends up in the emergency room five times in three weeks convinced that she is having a heart attack, even though each visit ends with the doctor assuring her, based on extensive (not to mention expensive) tests, that there is nothing wrong with her heart.

Is your anxiety causing you to make significant changes in the way you conduct your life? Do you find yourself catering to your anxiety, changing the things you do or the way you do them in an attempt to allay the unpleasant feelings? I am not suggesting, mind you, that there aren't very good reasons to make changes in your life. You would probably agree that it would make sense to cancel a romantic getaway weekend with your husband if your daughter had been running a fever for three days and you felt it was neither wise nor considerate to leave her with your elderly in-laws, or because the government had just issued a terror alert for the country you were planning to visit. But you might not agree that the actions of one of my patients made sense when, some years ago, she canceled an anniversary trip to a resort in Acapulco because a guidebook mentioned that there were numerous stray cats in the city. This woman was so phobic about cats that the thought of even glimpsing one was enough to make her forgo a vacation she had been planning for months and anticipating for years.

Similarly, you wouldn't question the anxiety you might feel about getting back onto a ski lift after the last ride up the mountain left you dangling in midair for thirty minutes, driving home alone at night after some thugs threw beer cans at your car window, or moments after the school nurse called to tell you that she was pretty sure the fall your child took on the playground didn't cause a concussion. Each of these scenarios presents circumstances under which a stable, well-adjusted person would have sufficient reason to feel anxious. But what if your anxiety didn't make sense to anyone, including you? What if it was so pervasive and chronic that it led you to make decisions that were detrimental to your career, your family, your social life, or all of the above?

That's what was happening to Melissa, who first came in for treatment in January 2003. She was thirty-two and worked as an assistant buyer of women's accessories for an upscale department store. She was married and the mother of a nine-year-old boy, and, except for a slight rash on her neck that reddened as she spoke, appeared to be the picture of health and self-confidence. I asked her what had brought her in to see me.

"My anxiety is running my life," she said. "I wake up with it and I go to sleep with it, although I usually don't stay asleep very long. I worry about everything. I mean *everything.* Sometimes I feel like there's a motor inside my body that just won't stop. And the craziest part is that most people look at me, my life, my job, my family, and think I don't have a care in the world!"

But they were wrong. Melissa fretted about her son, Cody (What if he lost the quarters she had given him to buy a snack? What if he went outside for recess without his jacket? What if he didn't eat enough for lunch? What if he ate too much for lunch? What if he didn't eat lunch at all?); her husband (What if he forgot to stop at the pharmacy and pick up his prescription? What if he had a car accident on the way to work? What if the pain in his back was something really serious?); her brother; her sister; and her parents (Did they remember what they were each supposed to bring to Christmas dinner? Would they allow enough time to get there in holiday traffic?); and the innumerable variables that constitute modern life (What if the airline canceled their flight and they missed her niece's confirmation? What if the pediatrician had vaccinated Cody with expired chicken pox vaccine and it didn't work—hadn't she just read something about that in a magazine?).

As I listened to Melissa talk, I was struck by how much insight she had regarding the things that were making her anxious and how aware she was that 95 percent of her anxiety was, as she put it, totally, undeniably irrational.

"Over the last six years I've been to four hospital emergency rooms and every '-ologist' you can think of," she said. She had seen not one but two cardiologists because she needed a second opinion after the first one said her heart palpitations were most likely anxiety-related, and then she consulted a neurologist who confirmed what she secretly believed: that both her frequent headaches and her difficulty concentrating on even menial tasks were due not to neurological problems but rather to stress. Some months earlier she had made an appointment with a gastroenterologist because a friend had been diagnosed with irritable bowel syndrome and Melissa thought perhaps she had it too since she had been having a lot of indigestion and upset stomachs (the doctor gave her some antacid samples, and, shortly afterward, the symptoms abated and had not returned). She had made an appointment with an endocrinologist for the week after she first came to see me and was hoping he would diagnose her with hyperthyroidism, which would at least explain her palpitations, skittishness, and fatigue.

Like many women with chronic, severe anxiety, Melissa had had the "million-dollar workup" and emerged with a clean bill of health among dozens of other bills. Ironically, during all the years of running from doctor to doctor she recalls only one who recommended she get psychiatric help, although after telling me this she backpedaled and admitted that others might have said the same thing, only she hadn't been ready to hear it.

"You've got to understand," she said, "I'm not making this stuff up—the headaches are real; the palpitations are real; the breathlessness is real. It's not just in my head."

"Isn't your head part of your body?" I asked.

Melissa and I discussed her symptoms, but before making a diagnosis and developing a treatment plan I needed more information: family history ("My mother and her mother were 'total worriers' "); caffeine intake (three to four cups of coffee a day); alcohol use ("None—I hate feeling out of control"); what types of situations made her tense, worried, or nervous ("Are you kidding? What doesn't make me nervous?"). Had her career been affected by it? ("Oh, yes; I should have lost the 'assistant' part of my title over two years ago, but I've taken so much sick leave that I haven't been promoted.") How about her relationship with her husband and son?

"That's probably what bothers me the most," she said. "Dan is so kind and patient, yet I snap at him for the most insignificant things. I'm so on edge all the time that it takes very little for me to get irritated. The same thing with Cody. One minute I'm smothering him, telling him he can't spend the night at a friend's house because he sneezed twice three hours ago, and the next minute I'm yelling at him because he's spending too much time alone playing video games. Let me tell you—I wouldn't want me for a mother or wife."

"How many days during the past six months would you say that you've experienced excessive anxiety and worry?" I asked.

"I would say . . ." Melissa closed her eyes briefly before answering. "You know, I can't remember a single day when I didn't feel anxious."

"Are there specific events or activities that are especially worrisome to you?" This unleashed a barrage of worries.

"I know Dan is faithful and I hate myself for thinking this, but sometimes when he comes home late I start wondering if maybe he's having an affair."

"What do you do when you have thoughts like that?"

"I'm embarrassed to admit this, but I call his cell phone and make up an excuse about why I'm calling. Then I start a conversation and try to find out exactly where he is."

"And when he tells you he's at the office, do you believe him?"

"Well, yes, but . . . this is so stupid, but even though I know that he is where he says he is, sometimes I start getting heart palpitations and I get all sweaty and my mind starts racing and thinking that he's not telling the truth."

"What do you do about it?"

"This is so embarrassing. I don't know if I can say it."

"That's fine; you don't have to unless you want to." She paused for a moment. Her face was flushed when she spoke again.

"Okay. Here goes. One time, I actually went online and looked up the extensions of everyone in Dan's department. Then I started calling around until this woman picked up the phone and I made up a phony name and asked if Dan was there. So she's like, 'You've got the wrong extension, but he's in his office so hold on and I'll transfer you—' and I hung up.

"And that's not all. One time I actually drove by his office to see if his car was still there. I put Cody in the car and drove around the back of the building until I saw his car, and then I drove home. Now, I realize this is totally crazy. I don't believe for a minute that my husband would cheat on me. He's never given me any reason to suspect he would do something like that. Intellectually, I know my anxiety is crazy. But I still can't stop the negative thoughts from creeping into my head and taking over my body."

"Are there other things you worry about that you know aren't really a danger to you?"

"Absolutely. I worry that we won't be able to save enough

money to send Cody to college. This is also crazy because Dan and I make decent salaries and we've already put quite a bit of money away for college. The other night I actually had what I think is a panic attack in the middle of the night. I'm lying there thinking, *What if something happens to Dan or me and we can't work anymore and we have to use Cody's college fund to pay the mortgage?* and on and on until I was a ball of sweat and had to get out of bed and walk around until I calmed down. And it's not as if Cody is leaving for college any time soon; he's only nine years old!"

Lack of sleep made Melissa exhausted all day, which then made her cranky and irritable all evening. When Dan recommended they go jogging together as an antianxiety activity, Melissa said she would give it a try. But their first time out she went a few blocks, became short of breath, and panicked, thinking she was having a heart attack. She hadn't put on her running shoes since.

Although Melissa felt beaten up by her anxiety, she was not clinically depressed. Sure, she said, there were times she felt she just couldn't stand feeling this way, but she never felt hopeless or so down that she couldn't function. I asked if she had ever had suicidal thoughts.

"No—never," she said. "Why would I want to kill myself? It's not that I don't want to be alive; it's just that it's so hard. At times I look around me and think, *I'm so much better off than most people: I have a good marriage, a wonderful kid, a nice house, and work I enjoy. So why does everyone else look so calm and relaxed and I always feel like I'm about to disintegrate?* You know, I'm so accustomed to feeling anxious that I can't even imagine what it would be like not to feel that way and to not always be worried about being worried."

It didn't take long for me to diagnose Melissa with generalized anxiety disorder (GAD). Unlike the everyday, normal anxiety we all feel from time to time, the physical and psychological symptoms associated with GAD are often so intense that they stop people from doing the very things they want and often love to do. In Melissa's case, her inability to concentrate, frequent headaches, and insomnia-related fatigue were interfering with her ability to keep up with the demands of her job and get promoted to a better one. That's what had finally driven her into my office (along with an event I'll describe later). She knew that her relentless anxiety and anxiety-related symptoms were different from those that many women feel while trying to juggle motherhood and career; she actually felt she had those areas well under control. I trusted Melissa when she described how helpful her husband was with their son; how well adjusted, mature, and independent Cody was; and how tolerant her boss was when she took time off for doctor visits or because she was too exhausted to work. Melissa's anxiety was not, as far as I could see, related to her lifestyle. She clearly had an anxiety disorder: GAD.

Laura, on the other hand, the twenty-eight-year-old daughter of a friend and the mother of three young children aged five, seven, and ten, has a lot to be anxious about. Any one of her family's challenges would drive many women to the brink of despair. Her seven-year-old suffers from autism, the nine-year-old has severe wheat allergies that frequently land her in the emergency room, and her husband was recently laid off from his job just as they were about to sign a contract on a new house.

Does Laura sometimes feel freaked out? Yes—often. When the phone rings and it's the school nurse, her heart starts racing in anticipation of learning that Jessica has eaten something she shouldn't have and gone into anaphylactic shock. Laura says she sometimes lies awake at night worrying how they will pay the mortgage on the old house—let alone afford to buy a new one—if her husband doesn't find work soon. Yet when I talk with Laura, I am consistently struck not only by how she is able to function as a mother and wife despite often feeling overwhelmed but also by how she takes concrete actions to alleviate her anxiety. She has prepared an instructional chart of what to do if Jessica has an allergy attack and given copies to Jessica's teachers, her friends' parents, the soccer coach, and the camp counselor. She started a local support group for parents of children with autism and begins each meeting with a five-minute breathing exercise she learned in a stress management seminar. She takes yoga classes three times a week, even, she says, if it means paying for a babysitter when her kids are off from school. "I used to think of yoga as a luxury, but I know now that it's a necessity," she says. "Those three hours a week of breathing, stretching, and just being still keep me from spinning out of control."

After not speaking with Laura for a few months, I bumped into her one evening during the Beltway sniper attacks of 2002. For three weeks that October, thousands of people living in the metropolitan Washington, D.C., area watched in horror as ordinary people just like them were gunned down, seemingly at random, as they filled their cars with gasoline, traversed shopping center parking lots, and did the things we all do every day without ever thinking our lives are about to end. Ten people were killed and three injured, including a thirteen-year-old boy who was shot and wounded as he arrived at his suburban Maryland middle school. The horror deepened. Some parents kept their children off the school bus, driving them instead and escorting them into the building; others kept them home from school altogether. Schools canceled recess and outdoor classes and went into lockdown mode. Two weeks later at the scene of the most recent shooting, the police found a handwritten letter, ostensibly from the snipers (it turned out there were two, a man and a teenage boy), whose postscript read, "Your children are not safe anywhere, at any time." The statement, which was widely publicized, chilled everyone who heard it. The fact that the shooters were captured the next day did not do much to contain the damage; the image of children being used for target practice slashed into our collective consciousness and stayed there.

During the twenty-two days of random rifle attacks, five million people in and around Washington, D.C., had to decide how to conduct their comings and goings and those of their families. Remember, too, that this happened just a year after the attacks of 9/11, in which one of the hijacked planes crashed into the Pentagon, killing a hundred people in the building and everyone on board. Among that horror, the anthrax attacks that began just one week later, and the Beltway shooting spree, people's emotions were jagged and raw and anxiety was running high. The sense of unseen, imminent danger was all anyone was talking about.

Now, I'm usually pretty good in crisis situations, but I have to admit that the Beltway shootings inspired some rather ridiculous behaviors on my part, such as the one I manifested when I went to the market to buy ingredients for a paella I was planning to cook for my husband that evening. As I drove around looking for a parking space, the news came over the radio that the sniper had shot a woman in a shopping center parking lot. The police chief was urging citizens to be extra-vigilant, especially when we were anywhere out in the open. I spied a vacant space adjacent to some bushes and pulled in, scanning the greenery to see if anyone was hiding there. I grabbed my purse, opened the door, and ran—yes, ran—as fast as I could into the market. Safely inside, I breathed deeply, found a cart, and proceeded to the seafood counter in relative calm. Some time later at the cash register, I glanced at the time stamped on my receipt and was surprised to see that I had spent forty-five minutes shopping—a lot longer than I had planned on. Armed with two grocery bags of shrimp, scallops, clams, saffron, and rice, I ventured into the parking lot and saw a broad, burly policeman standing smack in front of my car, shouting in my direction as I ran toward him. I began to panic—had they found the sniper hiding in the backseat? As I got closer, the policeman's eyes locked onto mine.

"Lady, do you realize that you left your door wide open with the keys in the ignition and the engine running?" I could feel the heat rise in my face. As manifestations of anxiety go, leaving your car unattended for forty-five minutes with the engine running is rather telling. I guess I was more than a little anxious.

Then there was the time I was asked to be a guest on a local cable television evening news show. It was about a week after the shootings began, and producers were creating special programs to help people deal with the stress and tension. I sat down and created a list of tips for dealing with the completely reasonable and utterly relentless anxiety that was making people tense, jittery, and convinced that their lives were in danger all the time. I prepared statistics so I could discuss the possibility of getting shot (whether it *could* happen) versus the probability of getting shot (the *likelihood* of it actually happening) and advice on how to talk to your children about what was going on and how to keep your own mind from playing out worst-case scenarios by focusing your attention on the present moment and not allowing it to wander.

I was about to leave the house to drive to the television station when *my* mind began to wander. Hadn't this sick and demented individual shown himself to thrive on notoriety? What could be more dramatic than attacking someone at a TV station when the entire city was glued to the news? And wasn't the station I was going to located behind a strip mall, next to a forested area? I asked my husband (who, as I mentioned earlier, worries a lot less than I do) to accompany me to the station. No problem. By the time we got there, the sun had gone down and it was pretty dark near the trees, where we were supposed to park. Ronnie wanted to let me off at the front door of the studio, but I insisted that I go with him to park the car—what if the sniper went after him after he dropped me off? So he parked the car and cut the engine. Before he could open his door, I grasped his hand and told him that someone on the radio had recommended that people not walk in a straight line when out in public because it was easier to aim and hit someone traveling in a predictable, linear pattern. Moments later there we were, zigging and zagging across the parking lot, huffing and puffing, my briefcase and purse flying, until I practically shoved us into the studio doorway. I was gasping for breath as the producer walked me onto the set and informed me that I would be on the air, live, in less than three minutes. They put me in a chair, smoothed my hair, and powdered my nose but didn't do anything for my racing heart and trembling legs (which, fortunately, were hidden under a desk). And thus, with a deep, cleansing breath and my most serene smile, I advised the Washington, D.C., cable television audience how important it was for us to remain calm.

It was in this fearful atmosphere that Laura and I ran into each other at the supermarket one night. Not surprisingly, the conversation began with "Great to see you, isn't this awful?" and progressed to "How are you and the kids handling this?" and then went on to "When do you think this nightmare will end?"

As we talked, Laura began to cry. She was having nightmares that the sniper was harming her family; she was following the news all day on the radio, television, and online; she was jumpy and edgy and could not quell the waves of anxiety that seized her throughout the day.

"I feel bad breaking down in front of you," she said. "You're a therapist, and the last thing you want to do on your off-hours is listen to an anxious person complain. But I feel so depleted. It's taking every ounce of control I have—and I don't have much left—to act normal and natural in front of the kids when I feel on the verge of hysteria inside."

I assured Laura that I was glad that she felt comfortable talking to me and that what she was experiencing was absolutely normal. I told her I believed that some of her anxiety was fueled by the fact that she was expending a great deal of energy on reassuring her children when she felt so frightened herself. She described how she and Frank had sat the children down together and explained that even though there were bad guys out there, their family was safe and Mommy and Daddy would protect everyone. She and Frank answered the children's questions as honestly as they could and played a cops-and-robbers game with them where they got the bad guys. And when their elementary school reopened after being closed for several days, Laura told Frank that, as jittery as she was, she wanted the kids to go back.

"The principal called all the parents, told us the school would be running in lockdown mode, and urged us to send our kids back in. I was tempted to keep them home, but I realized that doing that would be responding to my worries, not the actual likelihood of anything happening to them. I'm worried, all right, but I don't want to lay it on my kids. They're finally feeling safe and secure again, so why should I give them a reason to be anxious?"

Which brings me back to Melissa, who, after living for years with GAD and not knowing it, had finally come in for treatment. It was only two and a half months since the snipers had been captured, but she did not mention the attacks until the end of the session, when she said that seeing me on the (post-zigzag) cable TV show had caught her attention. She said that as she watched me reassure the audience that the anxiety they were experiencing was normal, it hit her like two tons of bricks that her anxiety was anything but normal. Yes, she felt all of the things I was talking about, but for her, that was just the beginning. When I described rational fear as fear that made some kind of sense, Melissa realized that the anxiety she experienced made no sense at all.

"Sure, the snipers freaked me out. But I was anxious long before they showed up, and I continued to feel that way long after they were captured. They'd been in custody for two weeks already, and I still couldn't bring myself to send Cody back to school. I told his teachers he was sick, got them to email me his assignments, and took some personal leave time from my job so I could stay home with him and avoid going outside myself. The truancy officer called but I hung up the phone, so they sent me a letter saying I had to provide a doctor's note, and then I became anxious about that. I made Dan call me from his cell phone on the way to work and after he got there so I'd know he was safe, and then he did the same thing in reverse on the way home. I'd talk to my friends and some of the people I worked with, and they were all able to get back to their old routines, but I was stuck. When Thanksgiving arrived and the school sent a social worker to the house, I knew I had to do something. So here I am."

Melissa had been paralyzed by her anxiety, much as we are in those nightmares where we're trying to flee a hideous monster but for some reason our legs won't move. Although she knew that the snipers were in jail (the progress of their legal travails and photos of them in prison jumpsuits were all over the media), she wasn't emotionally convinced that they wouldn't somehow show up at her son's school or along the road she took to work. Unlike someone who is clinically paranoid, Melissa did not have hallucinations or delusions of being followed or spied upon. But she was plagued by continuing insomnia, headaches, muscle tension, and spiraling "what if?" thoughts. She simply could not shake the anxiety.

If you were to spend any time at all with Laura and Melissa, I doubt that you would mistake either one for a laid-back, mellow kind of gal. Both cope with more anxiety on any given day than the average person. The difference between them is that Laura's anxiety varies in intensity and is rooted in rational concern about actual threats and hazards—her daughter's allergy, her son's autism, her husband's unemployment—while Melissa's anxiety is chronic, consistently excessive, and, for the most part, disconnected from any real threat. In other words, with some notable exceptions, Melissa's anxiety is almost entirely irrational.

That is the heart of all anxiety disorders: an inexplicable dread or fear that is just as irrational as it is uncontrollable. The sheer irrationality of the fear makes it even more frightening, as the person experiencing it cannot reason it away: it is simply, horrifyingly *there* and usually leads to either extreme distress or avoidance. In many cases, including Melissa's, extreme anxiety interferes mightily with a woman's everyday, moment-to-moment life, making it impossible for her to function fully in any of her numerous roles.

This is not always the case: if you were a kindergarten teacher in Des Moines with an elevator phobia, for instance, chances are it wouldn't affect your daily life as much as it would if you were an accountant with a job on the forty-second floor of a Chicago skyscraper. Which is not to say that an elevator-averse teacher doesn't have her own problems; it is merely to say that the degree to which anxiety affects a person varies according to both the severity of the anxiety and the circumstances of her life. And also to say that what a kindergarten teacher and an accountant with an elevator phobia have in common is that their fear doesn't make sense to either of them, yet they feel unable to control it. That's why we say they suffer from an anxiety disorder rather than from a normal fear.

EVERYDAY ANXIETY OR ANXIETY DISORDER?

So what exactly is an anxiety disorder? It's an umbrella term for a group of conditions that involve chronic, excessive, inexplicable anxiety that interferes with the way a person conducts his or her daily life. Under the umbrella are generalized anxiety disorder (GAD), panic disorder, phobias, social anxiety disorder, obsessive-compulsive disorder (OCD), and post-traumatic stress disorder (PTSD). Each of these conditions has a different constellation of symptoms, although some symptoms are common to several disorders. For instance, the pounding heart, shallow breathing, and excessive perspiration associated with panic disorder may also be familiar to someone who suffers from a specific phobia or social phobia. It is also common for a person to have more than one anxiety disorder, the varieties of which are as follows:

- As we established, Melissa is suffering from **generalized anxiety disorder (GAD)**. People who suffer from GAD are beset by persistent, excessive, and unrealistic worry that they are unable to control and that focuses on everyday things such as health, career, finances, relationships, and the security and well-being of their loved ones. GAD symptoms differ from those of the garden-variety worrier in that the worry associated with GAD is relentless and ongoing, feels impossible to control, and occurs on more days than not for a minimum of six months. The worries of GAD are accompanied by physical symptoms, especially restlessness, difficulty falling asleep and staying asleep, becoming easily fatigued, headaches, difficulty concentrating, irritability, muscle tension with resulting pain, abdominal upsets, and dizziness. Nearly seven million American adults, or 2 percent of the U.S. population, suffer from GAD, with women twice as likely as men to develop it. Women with GAD tend to develop the disorder younger than men and are more likely than men to have other mental health problems, such as depression.

- **Panic disorder** is characterized by recurrent, spontaneous, seemingly out-of-the-blue panic attacks, whose symptoms may include heart palpitations, sweating, trembling, shortness of breath or a feeling of choking, dizziness, chills, and hot flushes as well as fears of losing control, "going crazy" or dying, and feelings of imminent doom. Panic attacks manifest as abrupt onsets of intense terror that reach a peak within a few minutes. What differentiates someone with panic disorder from someone who experiences occasional panic attacks is the person's state of mind between the attacks: with panic disorder, an attack is typically followed by at least one month of persistent concern about having another attack, worry about the consequences of an attack (such as losing control or having a heart attack), and/or a major change in behavior related to the attacks.[3] Panic disorder affects twice as many women as men and is often accompanied by major depression. More than six million Americans—2.7 percent of the adult population—suffer from panic disorder.

- **Panic disorder with agoraphobia.** About one out of three people with panic disorder develops **agoraphobia,** an avoidance of places, typically open or public spaces, where one fears having a panic attack and being unable to immediately get to safety—for instance, when entering a theater or sports arena, waiting in line at the grocery store, or riding on public transportation. People with agoraphobia often start eliminating places they are willing to go as they relentlessly anticipate having a panic attack. In extreme cases, an agoraphobic's world gradually shrinks until he or she is too fearful to leave the house. Women with panic disorder are more likely than men to develop agoraphobia.

- **Specific or simple phobias** are characterized by irrational, involuntary fear reactions to particular objects, places, or situations. As with the example of the kindergarten teacher and the accountant with a fear of elevators, people who suffer from a specific phobia dread encountering ordinary, everyday situations or objects even though they know the dread is irrational. Someone with a phobia may even have a panic attack when confronted with a dreaded object or situation and thereafter be loath to go back for fear of having another panic attack. Oftentimes, it is anticipatory anxiety—the anxiety you feel when anticipating an event rather than the anxiety you feel when experiencing the event—that keeps a person from confronting something she has no realistic fear of (driving through a tunnel, petting her neighbor's kitten, riding on an escalator).

How can you tell the difference between a fear and a phobia? As stated earlier, if the aversion makes sense, it's probably a fear. If the aversion and accompanying feelings are irrational, it's probably a phobia. A person with a phobia fears the fear itself rather than the object of the fear and typically has difficulty defining exactly what he or she is afraid of. For example, if you ask someone with a fear of flying what she is afraid of, she will probably say "I'm afraid of crashing" or "I can't stand turbulence" or "I'm terrified we'll be hijacked by terrorists." Ask someone with a true flying phobia the same question, however, and she will probably say, "I don't know what I'm afraid of. What if I want to get off after we're airborne?" or "What if I have a panic attack on the plane and lose control and start running up and down the aisle like a madwoman?" or "What if I have a heart attack and die on the plane?" The "what if?" questions and fear of the feelings or the fear itself are characteristic of a phobia.

- **Social anxiety disorder,** also known as **social phobia,** is characterized by an intense fear of one or several social or performance situations in which the person is exposed to unfamiliar people and/or to possible scrutiny and judgment by others. Physical symptoms may include blushing, nausea, trembling, profuse sweating, and difficulty talking. Some people with social phobia are terrified of and make every effort to avoid specific situations requiring contact with others, such as speaking before an audience, making or receiving telephone calls, or signing their name in public. Others have a more generalized form of the disorder where they attempt to avoid or endure with great distress common, everyday social situations such as talking to authority figures (teachers, doctors, supervisors, police officers), being the center of attention at a meeting or social gathering, expressing disapproval of or disagreement with people they don't know well, or working while others are watching them. One of my patients, a twenty-year-old college freshman with the generalized type of social phobia, described his anxiety as affecting every aspect of his life and said, "The first thing I think about every morning when I first wake up is 'Who am I going to have to say hello to today?' "

Social phobia is the most common anxiety disorder, affecting fifteen million American adults. It's the third most common psychiatric disorder in the country after depression and substance abuse, and, interestingly, it is one of the few psychiatric disorders where men are more likely to seek treatment than women. We don't know for certain why this is the case, but one theory is that because it is less acceptable for men to be socially reticent than women, social anxiety poses more professional and personal difficulties for men, motivating them more to seek treatment.

- **Obsessive-compulsive disorder (OCD).** People who suffer from OCD are plagued by unwanted thoughts (obsessions) that intrude into their thinking. To ease the anxiety caused by these thoughts, they feel compelled to do certain things or perform ritualized acts (compulsions), all the while recognizing both the irrationality of their behavior and their inability to stop it. Common obsessions include constant, irrational worry about dirt, germs, or contamination; feelings that chaos will descend unless objects are positioned or a situation managed in a certain way; and apprehensiveness about disposing of items of little intrinsic value but that the person inexplicably feels she may someday need. Common compulsions include rituals associated with cleaning (repeated washing of hands or dusting and vacuuming); checking and rechecking (repeatedly making sure the door is locked, the iron unplugged, and the oven turned off before leaving the house); and hoarding (amassing excessive numbers of useful items such as dozens of bottles of shampoo or cases of soup or stockpiling useless items such as old newspapers and magazines or empty bottles and jars).
- **Post-traumatic stress disorder (PTSD)** is the one anxiety disorder that is rooted not in irrational fear but rather in an actual life-threatening event that the sufferer has either endured or witnessed. Once known as shell shock and used in reference to soldiers returning from battle with psychological disturbances, PTSD is diagnosed when a person is un-

able to recover from a traumatic experience (such as rape, physical abuse, or surviving a hurricane, tsunami, or earthquake) and continues to suffer from significant anxiety and depression for months and sometimes years afterward. People with PTSD often relive the traumatic event through nightmares and flashbacks and find it difficult if not impossible to concentrate, relax, or sleep undisturbed.

Whereas my purpose in this book is to explore everyday, normal anxiety, I have described the different anxiety disorders and will refer to them periodically because I want you to understand the difference between normal, healthy anxiety and the sort that is indicative of a medical condition that can and should be treated. Much of the last decade's most exciting work has focused on the disorders, and I believe we can infer a great deal about everyday anxiety from what science is teaching us about pathological anxiety. Many of my insights, musings, and conclusions, therefore, are founded on scientific research into anxiety disorders, and it is these that I will be sharing with you throughout this book.

With this in mind, I have included six questionnaires at the end of this chapter to help you evaluate your symptoms.

I am not suggesting that completing a questionnaire in this or any other book (or magazine) is a substitute for a competent professional evaluation. But I do believe that completing a well-designed questionnaire can stimulate and direct you to think about your situation in a clearheaded, logical way. Had Melissa completed these questionnaires, I believe she would have recognized her symptoms as those associated with GAD and sought help (and received relief) sooner than she did. As it happened, she was intelligent and self-aware and so was an excellent candidate for **cognitive-behavioral therapy (CBT)**, a mode of psychotherapy that attempts to help a person identify and modify the thoughts and behaviors that propagate the unrelenting anxiety associated with an anxiety disorder. CBT is founded on the belief that our feelings and behaviors—both desirable and undesirable—are rooted in our internal cognitions, or thoughts, rather than in external factors such as events, situations, or other people. The therapy encourages individuals to look at their thoughts as hypotheses that can be questioned and tested. Thus, when Melissa's mind was spiraling uncontrollably with thoughts of not having enough money to send her son to college, I asked her to separate the hard financial facts from her "what if?" catastrophic fantasies. When she began writing down all the reasons why her son's future was secure, she couldn't find a single rational reason why she should be worried and she was able to dismantle the spiral. This process of identifying and challenging irrational thoughts and replacing them with rational ones is the basis of CBT, which holds that most emotional and behavioral reactions are learned, thus making it possible to both unlearn unwanted reactions and learn new ones. As part of her therapy, in addition to teaching her how to identify and modify her faulty thinking, I encouraged Melissa to cut back on her caffeine intake, remove bedtime distractions (no television in the bedroom, for starters), and add relaxation techniques and routines to her daily schedule.

Many CBT techniques practiced by patients suffering from anxiety disorders are also effective at relieving everyday anxiety and stress. We'll get to those later on. For now, I invite you to find a quiet, private space and something to write with.

HOW MUCH ANXIETY IS TOO MUCH?

The questionnaires that follow are designed to help you determine if the anxiety, fear, or worry that bothers you is part of a normal, healthy reaction to everyday events or indicative of an anxiety disorder. As I've said, whereas filling out a questionnaire is not a substitute for getting a diagnosis from a health professional, it is a good place to start. If you answer yes to one or more of the questions in any of the questionnaires, you may want to take it with you to your physician or consider consulting a mental health professional.

As you go through the questions, you may identify your symptoms as characteristic of one or several disorders, or you may have symptoms that don't seem to fit neatly into any category. In either case, if your symptoms are causing you distress, I urge you to complete all six questionnaires, even if you think one or more of them describe symptoms that are unrelated to yours. If, for example, your chronic insomnia is soothed by vacuuming the house at two in the morning and you think this means you have obsessive-compulsive disorder, I want you to complete the questionnaires for social phobia, generalized anxiety disorder, and all the others as well. Why? Because you may have a preconceived notion about what your problem is, shape your thinking to conform to this notion, and, in so doing, overlook a symptom or series of symptoms that may reveal something else. And don't forget that if it turns out that you do indeed have an anxiety disorder, the good news is that it is treatable.

HOW CAN I TELL IF IT'S PANIC DISORDER?*

Are you troubled by:

❍ YES ❍ NO recurrent, unexpected "attacks" during which you are suddenly overcome by intense fear or discomfort, for no apparent reason?

* *Diagnostic and Statistical Manual of Mental Disorders, Fourth Edition* (*DSM-IV*) (Washington, D.C.: American Psychiatric Association, 1994). Questionnaire adapted from http://adaa.org/GettingHelp/SelfHelpTests/selftest_Panic.asp and used with permission of Anxiety Disorders Association of America.

During these attacks, do you experience any of these symptoms?

❍ YES ❍ NO pounding heart
❍ YES ❍ NO sweating
❍ YES ❍ NO trembling or shaking
❍ YES ❍ NO shortness of breath
❍ YES ❍ NO choking
❍ YES ❍ NO chest pain
❍ YES ❍ NO nausea or abdominal discomfort
❍ YES ❍ NO "jelly legs"
❍ YES ❍ NO dizziness
❍ YES ❍ NO feelings of unreality or being detached from yourself
❍ YES ❍ NO fear of dying
❍ YES ❍ NO numbness or tingling sensations
❍ YES ❍ NO chills or hot flushes

As a result of these attacks, do you:

❍ YES ❍ NO avoid places or situations where getting help or escaping might be difficult, such as in a crowd or standing in a line, or traveling in a bus, train, or car? (agoraphobia)

For at least one month following an attack, have you:

❍ YES ❍ NO felt persistent concern about having another one?
❍ YES ❍ NO worried about having a heart attack, losing control, or "going crazy"?
❍ YES ❍ NO changed your behavior because of the attack or the fear of having another one?

HOW CAN I TELL IF IT'S A PHOBIA?*

Are you troubled by:

❍ YES ❍ NO persistent and unreasonable fear of an object, place, or situation, such as flying, heights, animals, blood, etc.?

❍ YES ❍ NO avoidance of specific places or situations, such as elevators, tunnels, bridges, or escalators?

❍ YES ❍ NO severe anxiety responses or panic attacks when you're exposed to the feared object, place, or situation?

❍ YES ❍ NO an awareness that your fear is excessive or unreasonable?

HOW CAN I TELL IF IT'S SOCIAL ANXIETY DISORDER (ALSO KNOWN AS SOCIAL PHOBIA)?†

Are you troubled by:

❍ YES ❍ NO intense and persistent fear and/or avoidance of social situations in which you imagine people might judge you?

❍ YES ❍ NO fear that you will be humiliated by your actions?

❍ YES ❍ NO fear that people will notice that you are blushing, sweating, trembling, or showing other signs of anxiety?

* *Diagnostic and Statistical Manual of Mental Disorders, Fourth Edition* (*DSM-IV*) (Washington, D.C.: American Psychiatric Association, 1994). Questionnaire adapted from http://adaa.org/GettingHelp/SelfHelpTests/selftest_specialpho.asp and used with permission of Anxiety Disorders Association of America.

† *Diagnostic and Statistical Manual of Mental Disorders, Fourth Edition* (*DSM-IV*) (Washington, D.C.: American Psychiatric Association, 1994). Questionnaire adapted from http://adaa.org/GettingHelp/SelfHelpTests/selftest_socialpho.asp and used with permission of Anxiety Disorders Association of America.

❍ YES ❍ NO severe anxiety responses or panic attacks when you're exposed to the feared situation?

❍ YES ❍ NO knowing that your fear is excessive or unreasonable?

COULD IT BE OCD (OBSESSIVE-COMPULSIVE DISORDER)?*

❍ YES ❍ NO Do you have unwanted ideas, images, or impulses that seem silly, nasty, or horrible?

❍ YES ❍ NO Do you worry excessively about dirt, germs, or chemicals?

❍ YES ❍ NO Are you constantly worried that something bad will happen because you forgot to do something important, such as lock the front door or turn off appliances?

❍ YES ❍ NO Are you afraid you will act or speak aggressively when you don't mean to?

❍ YES ❍ NO Do you avoid situations or people you fear you will hurt by speaking or acting aggressively?

❍ YES ❍ NO Are you always afraid you will lose something of importance?

❍ YES ❍ NO Are there things you feel you must do excessively or thoughts you must think repeatedly to feel comfortable or ease anxiety?

❍ YES ❍ NO Do you wash yourself or things around you excessively?

* W. K. Goodman, L. H. Price, et al., "The Yale-Brown Obsessive Compulsive Scale (Y-BOCS): Part 1. Development, Use and Reliability," *Archives of General Psychiatry* 46 (1989):1006–1011; *Diagnostic and Statistical Manual of Mental Disorders, Fourth Edition* (*DSM-IV*) (Washington, D.C.: American Psychiatric Association, 1994). Questionnaire adapted from http://adaa.org/GettingHelp/SelfHelpTests/selftest_OCD.asp and used with permission of Anxiety Disorders Association of America.

❍ YES ❍ NO Do you have to check things over and over or repeat them many times to be sure they are done properly?

❍ YES ❍ NO Do you keep many useless things because you feel that you cannot throw them away?

❍ YES ❍ NO Are you aware that your obsessions and/or compulsions are excessive or unreasonable?

❍ YES ❍ NO Do your obsessions or compulsions distress you, consume more than an hour of your time every day, or interfere significantly with your normal routine, professional and/or academic functioning, or social relationships?

HOW CAN I TELL IF IT'S GAD (GENERALIZED ANXIETY DISORDER)?*

Are you troubled by:

❍ YES ❍ NO excessive worry, occurring more days than not, for at least six months?

❍ YES ❍ NO unreasonable worry about a number of events or activities, such as work, school, and/or health?

❍ YES ❍ NO an inability to control the worry?

Are you bothered by at least three of the following symptoms?

❍ YES ❍ NO restlessness, feeling keyed up or on edge

❍ YES ❍ NO becoming easily fatigued

❍ YES ❍ NO problems concentrating

* *Diagnostic and Statistical Manual of Mental Disorders, Fourth Edition* (*DSM-IV*) (Washington, D.C.: American Psychiatric Association, 1994). Questionnaire adapted from http://adaa.org/GettingHelp/SelfHelpTests/selftest_GAD.asp and used with permission of Anxiety Disorders Association of America.

❍ YES ❍ NO irritability
❍ YES ❍ NO muscle tension
❍ YES ❍ NO trouble falling asleep or staying asleep, or restless and unsatisfying sleep

HOW CAN I TELL IF IT'S PTSD (POST-TRAUMATIC STRESS DISORDER)?*

❍ YES ❍ NO Have you experienced or witnessed a life-threatening event that caused you to feel intense fear, helplessness, or horror?

Do you reexperience the event in at least one of the following ways?

❍ YES ❍ NO repeated, distressing memories and/or dreams
❍ YES ❍ NO acting or feeling as if the event were happening again (flashbacks or a sense of reliving the event)
❍ YES ❍ NO intense physical and/or emotional distress when you are exposed to things that remind you of the event

Do you avoid reminders of the event and feel numb, compared to the way you felt before the event, in three or more of the following ways?

❍ YES ❍ NO avoiding thoughts, feelings, or conversations about it
❍ YES ❍ NO avoiding activities, places, or people who remind you of it
❍ YES ❍ NO blanking out on important parts of it

* *Diagnostic and Statistical Manual of Mental Disorders, Fourth Edition* (*DSM-IV*) (Washington, D.C.: American Psychiatric Association, 1994). Questionnaire adapted from http://adaa.org/GettingHelp/SelfHelpTests/selftest_PTSD.asp and used with permission of Anxiety Disorders Association of America.

❍ YES ❍ NO losing interest in activities that were once important to you
❍ YES ❍ NO feeling detached from other people
❍ YES ❍ NO feeling your range of emotions is restricted
❍ YES ❍ NO sensing that your future has shrunk (for example, you don't expect to have a career, marriage, children, or normal life span)

Are you troubled by two or more of the following symptoms?

❍ YES ❍ NO sleeping problems
❍ YES ❍ NO irritability or outbursts of anger
❍ YES ❍ NO problems concentrating
❍ YES ❍ NO feeling on guard or on alert
❍ YES ❍ NO an exaggerated startle response

Do your symptoms interfere with your daily life?

❍ YES ❍ NO

Have your symptons lasted for at least one month?

❍ YES ❍ NO

three

IT'S NOT JUST IN YOUR HEAD— IT'S IN YOUR BRAIN (AND THE REST OF YOUR BODY, TOO)

Ten years ago a producer from the *Today* show invited me to do a segment on the latest research into women and anxiety disorders. I had been on the show a few years earlier, when my first book had come out, and had been both surprised and gratified by the response to the show. Moments after it aired, the switchboard at the Anxiety Disorders Association of America lit up with calls from people all over the country asking for more information about anxiety, and in the weeks that followed letters poured in from people saying they were glad to have a name for what they were experiencing and how, after years of secrecy, shame, and desperation, they finally had hope that they might recover.

So I was excited when *Today* invited me on again, and I started thinking about how I might organize the information I wanted to get across. It soon became clear to me that I had treated a diverse array of women and had an abundance of information to share. It also became clear that the information I had was anecdotal, not scientific. Yes, I could talk for hours about women who had overcome paralyzing bouts of anxiety, but there were very few studies I could cite that supported, with hard data, the experiences my patients were talking about. The Internet was not yet well developed, and what data there was I had gleaned from research papers my colleagues had sent me. As I leafed through my files, I also realized that there was very little research that focused on women.

Yet I had data; it was right there in my patients' files. I had treated women with panic disorder whose symptoms abated when they became pregnant. And I had treated other women who first came in for therapy after they got pregnant because, out of the blue, they developed symptoms of obsessive-compulsive disorder when their pregnancies began. I pictured myself sitting with Katie Couric and talking passionately about these women, and then I pictured Katie Couric asking me about the research and me sitting there telling her that we didn't really have data to back up what I was seeing in my practice.

My heart fell, but I knew what I had to do. I picked up the phone, called the producer, and told him with genuine regret that I had to decline the invitation. My family and friends thought I was crazy to turn down the *Today* show, and a part of me agreed with them. But a bigger part of me was heartened by the response of my colleagues, who praised me for declining an opportunity to broadcast anecdotal evidence that, however intriguing, had no scientific support.

That event galvanized me: a hugely popular morning television show was ready, willing, and eager to air a segment on women and anxiety disorders, and there wasn't enough research to back up an interview. I knew what I had to do. I started talking with my colleagues to learn who was doing what, so we could figure out what wasn't being done and start getting it done.

Five years later, in 2004, my ADAA colleagues and I convened our first scientific meeting devoted to women and anxiety disorders. Finally, there was enough science to bring together some of the top researchers in the country and ask them: What do we know about anxiety disorders and women? What don't we know? What connection exists between anxiety and biochemistry—specifically, a woman's body chemistry? How much of what we call anxiety is intangible emotion, and how much is a measurable, chemical reaction? In short, how is it that the brain, that colossus of logic and rationality, is still vulnerable to unreasonable, inexplicable bouts of anxiety?

WHAT WAS I THINKING?

It isn't news that emotions frequently overrule reason; the media abound with stories of people acting in ways that defy the existence of their brains: the spurned lover who stalks and murders the woman he claims to adore; the disgruntled employee who returns to his office and shoots half a dozen coworkers before turning the gun on himself. We can all relate, if with less drama and violence: Who among us hasn't hurled a nasty remark at someone we love and wondered, as the words still vibrated in the air, Why did I say that? What was I thinking? (We weren't.) Or ordered a gooey, rich dessert that our rational mind told us would make us feel sick and loathe ourselves (which it did), just because we wanted it so badly when we saw it on the menu?

Or take my friend Iris, an American journalist based in Europe who happened to be in town some time ago. Strolling the glittering cosmetics concourse in a tony department store, we were approached by two sleek-skinned, white-coated beauties who persuaded us to let them demonstrate, on our not-so-sleek middle-aged faces, the latest makeup stylings. After a dusting of eye shadow and a dollop of lipstick, I was off to the shoe department, leaving Iris to catch up with me later. Two pairs of boots and six pairs of pantyhose later, I found her beside me sporting a small, shiny shopping bag, a full cosmetic makeover, and a dubious expression.

"What's the matter?" I asked. "Don't you like your makeup?"

"I'd better like it," she said, "because I just spent over three hundred bucks on it." She jiggled the shopping bag, which looked too small to hold three hundred dollars' worth of anything that wasn't measured in carats. "It's not a matter of whether I like it or not," she said. "It's that I need more makeup like a hole in the head."

"So why did you buy it?"

"How could I *not* buy it? She spent an hour on me and told me how great I looked, and then all the other white coats came over and told me how great I looked. I would have felt like a complete worm if I didn't buy anything."

Iris is probably the best-traveled, worldliest, most intrepid person I know. She has reported from hot zones around the world and does not have any trouble asserting herself. Yet she allowed her emotions (worry about appearing stingy and ungrateful) to overrule her reason (knowing she did not need more cosmetics) and shelled out a lot of money for several ounces of powders, pencils, and emollients that were no better than the ones she already owned and that, in any case, she would probably never use.

Why, then, are our emotions—anxiety prominently among them—so often able to override our ability to think clearly? I had my own run-in with this phenomenon just a few days ago. For the past five years, I've been working out with a trainer early in the morning several times a week. When I started, both my mother and father were in declining health, and between taking care of them, working full-time, traveling, and dealing with my own health issues, I was wracked with stress and knew it was important for me to maintain a regular exercise regimen (which was why I decided to hire a trainer: if I knew Brian was waiting for me at the gym, I couldn't make up an excuse and not go). On several occasions, my cell phone had rung during a workout and it had been one of my parents' caretakers telling me either that my father was disoriented and might be having another stroke or that my mother, who had cancer, was taking a turn for the worse. I rarely received any calls at 7:00 A.M. other than those that related to my parents, so my heart would race wildly whenever the phone rang and I would bolt to answer it.

Just a few days ago, there I was at half past seven in the morning, lifting 130 pounds on the assisted pull-up machine with Brian urging me on, when my cell phone rang. My heart leapt and so did I, off the machine and toward my phone, when I realized that I had let go of the weight, which had plunged downward and would have crushed Brian's hand had it not been for a safety feature on the apparatus. I was (and still am) horrified at how close I came to severely injuring another person and stunned at how even now, two years after my mother passed away, and despite knowing that my father is well tended by the staff at the assisted-living facility where he lives, my reaction was no different from what it was five years ago. I am, of course, fully aware that my mother is gone and that my father, who is nearly ninety as I write this, is of an age where every day I have him is a blessing.* Still, my response remained entirely automatic, distilled of pure emotion and panic, with no thought tempering my actions. It was only after I had acted that I understood what I had done and the terrible consequences that might have ensued.

Why did this happen? Why are our rational minds sometimes utterly overruled by irrational emotions?

Because the brain is hardwired to respond that way. We have known for some time that when a person perceives a threat to him- or herself (or, in some cases, to someone else), the body rapidly undergoes a set of physiological changes known as the fight-or-flight response (physicians and scientists tend to refer to it as the stress response). It's the centerpiece of each person's bodily homeland security system, evolved over thousands of years as humans learned either to defend themselves against predators or perish. Although saber-toothed cats seldom invade our hearths today, we remain amply equipped, as do other mammals, to respond swiftly when we feel we're in danger; we just respond to

* Sadly, my father passed away after the draft of this book was completed.

different signals now than we did then. You know what I'm talking about: the phone rings at four in the morning, and you're wide awake with your heart in your throat; you're summoned to the boss's office ASAP, and your pulse starts racing; you return home to find a squad car parked in front of your house, and you're on the verge of hyperventilating by the time you learn that the police are visiting not you but the people next door. In each of these scenarios, the perception of a threat causes your brain to activate a series of chemical reactions that prepare your body to perform at peak levels so it can either fight a predator or flee it. Never mind that the alleged predator may be nothing more than some poor guy who dialed a wrong number; as far as your brain is concerned, a shrill ring at 4:00 A.M. means trouble, and it's your brain's mission to prepare you to cope with it.

It does this with breathtaking efficiency by translating sensory signals—what we see, hear, smell, feel, and taste—into thoughts: it looks like a small animal scurrying in front of the car! . . . but it's actually a dry leaf skittering across the road; it sounds like a volley of gunfire next door! . . . but it's actually the neighbors setting off fireworks. We used to think that the body responded based on a coherent analysis—not mouse but leaf, not gunfire but fireworks—of the sensory signals. But research by Joseph LeDoux, Ph.D., at New York University shows that the brain catalyzes the body to respond to sensory input even before it analyzes the input, inspiring an instantaneous emotional response before a more nuanced, analytical one.[1] The notion that we seem to have no choice but to respond emotionally (irrationally) before we respond cerebrally (rationally) has fascinating implications for the way we look at anxiety as well as for the way we look at the brain.

Before we further explore the brain and its renowned fight-or-flight response, I should mention a relatively new and captivating model of how people—especially women—respond to stress. The model suggests that when women are confronted with a threat, our repertoire of responses includes not only fighting or fleeing but also doing something rather different: digging in, protecting our young, and fortifying ourselves by bonding with others. Dubbed the "tend-and-befriend" response by Shelley E. Taylor, Ph.D., who developed the model with her colleagues at the University of California, Los Angeles, this new way of looking at stress-related behaviors provides a fresh perspective on how women's response to stress may differ from men's.

Dr. Taylor's team began looking more closely at stress response research when they realized that, until fairly recently, almost all such research had been conducted on men. They reviewed the existing scientific literature and deduced that, although both women and men typically respond to an immediate, intense threat by fighting or fleeing, "a stress response geared toward aggressing or fleeing may be somewhat adaptive for males but it may not address the different challenges faced by females, especially those challenges that arise from maternal investment in offspring."[2] In other words, fighting and fleeing is sometimes more representative of guy behavior than gal behavior. Their theory is that women's responses to stress have evolved not only to overcome or flee it but also to maximize the chances of their own survival and that of their children. To this end, Dr. Taylor's team concluded that women typically tend their young and befriend other adults, often women, to mitigate and manage stress and reduce the risk of harm.

Whereas research into tending and befriending behaviors is relatively new, the data is supported by what we all know: that when a woman is struggling with a problem and feeling stressed out, chances are good that she will phone, email, or, best of all, get together with her sister, mother, friend, or group of friends to unburden herself, talk things through, and get support. These behaviors may not be new, but what is new is the knowledge that they are about a lot more than socializing: they are, in fact, a vital component of woman's stress-management mechanism. They are also, Dr. Taylor believes, possibly moderated by the hormone oxytocin, whose levels rise greatly during pregnancy and which seems to exert a calming effect (hence the fabled radiance and serenity of women when they are with child; you can read more about oxytocin later in this chapter).[3]

The bottom line is, for women and men, that both anxiety and our responses to it are hardwired, to a greater or lesser extent, into our heads—into our brains, to be precise—wherein a cascade of chemicals causes us to react in reassuringly familiar or bizarrely unpredictable ways. To give you an idea of how it works, I shall re-create the vivid scenario created by Dr. LeDoux of NYU, which is better than any I could come up with on my own.[4]

Imagine it's a clear, crisp day and you're walking through the woods. Approaching a log in the path, you see a snake directly beyond it, just where your foot would land were you to step over the log. Your eyes take in the information—brown, coiled, sinuous—and transmit the visual signals to the thalamus, a mass of nuclei deep within the brain that is believed to translate and transmit sensory signals to other parts of the brain. According to LeDoux, a portion of the thalamus then sends unrefined and, in his words, almost archetypal information directly to the amygdala, a small, almond-shaped portion of the brain that controls emotional responses.[5] The transmission of this information directly to the amygdala, the feeling part of the brain, prompts the brain to start responding to the possible danger posed by a brown, sinuous object, which might be a snake but might also be part of a tree branch, a length of rope, or some other harmless entity such as a belt, which you might encounter were you strolling in your closet instead of the woods. At the same time, the thalamus is sending information to the neocortex, which is able to decipher more details about the object than either the thalamus or the amygdala acting alone. The neocortex registers detailed information about the stimulus and integrates supplementary information about context to come up with an accurate interpretation—it's a snake, not a branch or a rope or a belt (this cortical circuit also establishes a belt as incongruous in the woods). Detailed analysis complete, the neocortex forwards refined information to the amygdala.

LeDoux points out that although the neocortex's information is more detailed than the thalamus's, it takes longer to reach the amygdala. The direct thalamus-to-amygdala transmission, however unrefined, LeDoux emphasizes, enables the amygdala to respond a split second faster to a potential threat, perhaps meaning the difference between life and death.

In that split second, the brain juices the body with chemicals: the hypothalamus (located below the thalamus and just above the brain stem) secretes corticotropin-releasing* hormone, or CRH, which makes its way to the pituitary gland, which dwells at the base of the brain. When it arrives, CRH stimulates the pituitary to secrete adrenocorticotropin hormone, or ACTH, into the bloodstream, which in turn stimulates the adrenal glands (these are not in the brain but rather perched atop the kidneys) to produce cortisol, a steroid stress hormone.[6]

Cortisol's effects are swift and dramatic: it inhibits the immune response, preventing tissue damage by reducing the body's potential for inflammation; adjusts metabolic functions to aid and abet fighting or fleeing or a combination of the two (cortisol is a glucocorticoid, a class of substances released during stress that help maintain blood glucose to sustain bodily energy); makes the heart contract faster and more intensely; and sharpens the senses by sensitizing blood vessels to the effects of norepinephrine (also known as noradrenaline).[7]

Which is why, for instance, a woman may feel electrified by an adrenaline rush when she senses a large presence standing behind her in the kitchen—until the thinking part of her brain informs her that the presence is her husband or son or boyfriend or roommate and not an intruder. It takes only a fraction of a second for her to recognize the figure as friend, not foe, and to infer that he either just arrived home or padded in from the other room in his stocking feet without her hearing him. But for a freaky split sec-

* I have encountered two spellings: corticotro*ph*in and corticotro*p*in; I am using the latter, following the example of *The New England Journal of Medicine.*

ond the rational, thinking part of her brain, the neocortex, is overruled by the emotional, feeling part, the amygdala, which detects a looming presence that could mean danger.

Once the looming presence is reframed as the adorable big lug she lives with, she shrieks, "Ooh, you scared me!," admonishes him not sneak up on her like that (to which he almost certainly replies that he didn't mean to), and returns to washing dishes, sautéing shallots, or whatever she was doing before she got spooked. Her pulse slows down, her breathing returns to normal, and her muscles relax as norepinephrine and cortisol recede to normal levels.

That's how it's supposed to work. In a healthy person, once the stressful moment passes, the fight-or-flight response is defused, the immune system restored to its prestress operating level and the body to a state of equilibrium.[8]

But it doesn't always work that way. When people live in chronically stressful circumstances or are beset by excessive anxiety, their stress hormones may never get a chance to recede to noncrisis levels. The result is that they live in a long-term low-level fight-or-flight state, with chronically elevated cortisol levels inhibiting the immune response for days, weeks, months, and even years, leaving them more vulnerable to infection and disease. This is no small issue: studies of people caring for chronically ill loved ones show that ongoing stress and anxiety contribute to a host of serious medical problems, including premature fraying of the chromosomes.[9]

So what should we do—develop drugs to lower our cortisol levels as we do our cholesterol count? Alas, it's not that simple: as do many other biochemicals, cortisol serves numerous functions, and inhibiting the immune response is only one of them. In fact, new studies show that cortisol and other glucocorticoids seem to protect us from some negative effects of anxiety. A 2006 Swiss study of people with phobias found that doses of cortisol taken by mouth eased the symptoms of spider phobia (a related study found that cortisone, another glucocorticoid, eased social phobia symptoms),[10] and a 2007 German study of forty-four healthy, nonphobic young women found that similarly administered doses of cortisol seemed to soften the negative effects of performing a series of anxiety-provoking tasks.[11] The researchers concluded that supplementary doses of cortisol seem to protect people from some of the onerous and immediate effects of anxiety and stress.

So is cortisol good or bad? Both or neither? What should we take away from all this?

First, that biology is seldom as simple as we would like it to be. Second, that as with many other biochemicals, cortisol's effects are intended to last only as long as the stress they are meant to deal with, and when cortisol continues to be produced after the stress ends, the cumulative effects lead to wear and tear on the body.

And third, that hormones are powerful agents in both the body's chemical reaction to anxiety and our experience of it. Which brings us to the mother of all hormones: estrogen.

WOMEN, ESTROGEN, AND ANXIETY

Scientists have recently begun to look at the relationship between women's anxiety and the life cycle (as in reproduction, not the workout machine), and, as I mentioned in Chapter 1, there is mounting evidence to support what a lot of us have long suspected: that our hormones have a major effect on when and how intensely we experience anxiety. Researchers have found, for example, that female mice that have been treated with estrogen over a long period of time exhibit more intense anxietylike behaviors than do female mice that have not been treated with estrogen, the inference being that estrogen just might intensify fear responses in human females as well.[12]

There's also evidence that estrogen increases a woman's ability to detect fear responses in others and regulates this ability according to where she is in her menstrual cycle. In a study of college students, researchers found that the young women's ability to correctly read other people's faces fluctuated both with the emotion being displayed and where they were in their cycles. Specifically, the students were a lot better at recognizing fear in other people's faces when they were ovulating—that is, when estrogen levels are highest—than they were when they were menstruating, when estrogen levels are lowest.[13]

Why should this be the case? From an evolutionary standpoint, it makes sense: heightened perceptive powers stand a woman in good stead. This is especially true when she is fertile and capable of creating new life: if she can discern something about a guy from his face, she can make a better decision about whether or not she wants to get acquainted with the rest of him and carry his offspring. From a cavewoman's perspective, when a guy approaches, club in hand, it would be useful to be able to judge whether he was likely to ignore her, ask her for food, want to mate with her, or whack her over the head, forever robbing posterity of her unique genetic legacy. And if she is astute enough to read fear in his face—or the face of anyone else who happens to be nearby, male or female—she might be warned of approaching danger in enough time to save her skin. Which, of course, is just as useful a trait today as it was several millennia ago.

ANXIETY AND GENDER DIFFERENCES

We know that estrogen seems to affect and intensify anxiety in women, and we know that women's anxiety seems to vary according to where they are in their reproductive lives. So it follows that fluctuating estrogen levels account for women's fluctuating levels of anxiety, right?

Maybe. Probably. But maybe not entirely. Should you find me frustratingly namby-pamby about this, allow me to explain myself. The research in this field is expanding and deepening rapidly, and it's easy to want the various findings to coalesce into a tidy, harmonious whole. But it is just too soon to toss a tiara onto estrogen's mighty head and crown her queen of the anxiety court. It's like being invited onto the *Today* show: as much as you may want to do it, you have to discipline yourself to acknowledge what you don't know as well as celebrate what you do know. One conclusion we drew from the 2004 ADAA conference was that the effect of women's reproductive hormones on anxiety is an understudied area that would benefit from more collaboration among researchers. So although it looks as if estrogen does play a major role in women's experience of anxiety, we lack the data at this point to state definitively what its role is, how it does what it does, and why it does what it does. Scientists agree, in fact, that it is unlikely that a single factor or mechanism is liable for all the differences between women's and men's experience of anxiety.[14] For example, there is also evidence that progesterone, a steroid hormone involved in the menstrual cycle and pregnancy, is also involved in modulating anxiety. By the time you read this, there will be more data about progesterone's effects on anxiety, but right now, a lot of what we know is theoretical.

Still, we do know that women tend to be more anxious than men and are twice as likely as men to develop panic disorder, specific phobia, or generalized anxiety disorder; they are also more likely than men to develop post-traumatic stress disorder (until age fifty, when the risk factor for women and men evens out). The only anxiety disorders that affect men and women with similar frequency are obsessive-compulsive disorder and social anxiety disorder. In fact, obsessive-compulsive disorder is more common in boys than girls in the years before puberty and tends not to manifest in women until they reach adulthood.[15]

For most anxiety disorders, however, the gender difference shows up as early as age six, when girls are twice as likely as boys to have one. This is significant, because the effects of an anxiety disorder transcend the girlhood years, frequently complicating a woman's other medical conditions later in life. Anxiety also commonly occurs along with depression: Australian researchers have found that women who develop depression in adulthood are more likely than not to have also suffered from an anxiety disorder in childhood.[16] What this means, of course, is that we must take manifestations of anxiety in young girls very seriously, as it could develop into serious health problems later in life.

ANXIETY AND THE FEMALE LIFE CYCLE

Here, then, is an overview of what we know about gender differences in the experience of anxiety:

- **Women are at (much) greater risk than men.** Thirty-one percent of women will develop some sort of anxiety disorder at some point in their lives, compared to 19 percent of men. Which means, if you're fond of statistics, that a girl is 85 percent more likely than her brother to develop an anxiety disorder at some point in her life.
- **Fluctuating hormones seem to modulate anxiety.** Women tend to experience more anxiety symptoms during the fertile phase of their menstrual cycles; pregnancy seems to keep the symptoms of some anxiety disorders at bay while hastening the appearance of others; and the menopausal transition is notorious for causing anxiety in women who never had problems with it before.
- **Society and culture don't help.** Along with the hormonal ups and downs that occur throughout a woman's life are anxiety-inducing messages from society and popular culture informing her that, to be sexually desirable, she must grow breasts during puberty (and maintain them in pubescent perfection for the rest of her life), get married and have kids in young womanhood, be a perfect wife and mother for unspecified decades, and stay nubile and sexy throughout the menopausal transition, menopause, and beyond.

Here is what we know about how anxiety manifests and changes across the stages of a woman's life:

- **Childhood.** Many women and men who suffer from an anxiety disorder can trace its beginnings back to childhood. Moreover, the age of onset seems to be the same for both sexes: little girls don't manifest anxiety any earlier or later than do little boys. But that changes by age six, when girls are twice as likely as boys to have an anxiety disorder. We are not sure of why this is, but it suggests an early biological difference in risk between males and females.[17]
- **Adolescence and the start of menstruation (menarche).** The hormones that flood a girl's system when she starts menstruating can change both the way she feels and the way she perceives the world—for a few days each month, at least. They also affect anxiety, in some cases prompting it to emerge for the first time: both obsessive-compulsive disorder and post-traumatic stress disorder become more common among girls when they hit puberty.
  - **Obsessive-compulsive disorder.** OCD is more common in boys than girls until adolescence, when a substantially higher number of girls start manifesting OCD symptoms. Researchers believe the flood of reproductive hormones in girls' systems accounts for the upsurge. This is consistent with the fact that the luteal and late-luteal phases of the menstrual cycle—that is, when a woman is ovulating and most fertile—are associated with both the appearance and intensification of OCD symptoms. In fact, even women who don't have OCD are known to act a bit as if they do during the fertile phase of their cycle: a study of college students who did not have OCD found they exhibited more OCD-like behaviors—such as cleaning things they didn't usually clean or cleaning things that were already clean—during the luteal phase than at any other time during their menstrual cycle.[18] (Next time you get an urge to clean out the garage at one in the morning, check the calendar—you might just be ovulating.)

- **Post-traumatic stress disorder.** Though women and men are exposed to traumatic events at equal rates across their lifetimes, some data suggest that females experience trauma earlier as a result of sexual assault: in six of ten forcible rapes of females, the victim is eighteen years old or younger; a third of these are children aged eleven and younger.[19]

  By adolescence, teenage girls are at the same risk of developing PTSD as adult women and five to six times more likely to develop PTSD than their male classmates. We don't know for certain why this is the case, but one theory is that the bafflements of female adolescence—shaky self-esteem, erosion of academic self-confidence, the intensity and volatility of friendships with other girls, and all-consuming relationships with romantic partners—overwhelm many girls' ability to cope and leave them vulnerable to the disorder. Another component of the increased prevalence of PTSD among teenage girls may be sexual assault, as noted above. Adolescent girls who develop PTSD are at greater risk of depression and thoughts of suicide, academic failure, run-ins with the law, alcohol and drug abuse, and generally diminished health.[20] Recent findings also suggest that experiencing trauma earlier in life may place a woman at risk for developing premenstrual dysphoric disorder (see below).

  Does this mean that every teenage girl who has a traumatic experience will develop PTSD and a raft of other problems? Absolutely not. Most people rebound from trauma and are able to heal. Research into why some people can do this and others cannot is still in its infancy.

- **Premenstrual dysphoric disorder (PMDD).** We have all heard, talked, and joked about premenstrual syndrome (PMS), an undefined conglomeration of symptoms that often appear prior to menstruation. There is also a specific medical disorder associated with menstruation known as premenstrual dysphoric disorder (dysphoria denotes a state of malaise, unhappiness, or lack of well-being), which the *Diagnostic and Statistical Manual of Mental Disorders, Fourth Edition* (*DSM-IV*) defines as the presence of at least five of eleven symptoms, with at least one of them being anxiety, depressed mood, moodiness, or irritability. The other symptoms include fatigue, reduced ability to concentrate, increased appetite, decreased interest in typical activities, change in sleep patterns, feeling overwhelmed or out of control, and physical symptoms such as abdominal cramping and breast tenderness.

When an adolescent consistently exhibits or complains of uncomfortable premenstrual symptoms, it is worth having a doctor determine whether she is experiencing garden-variety discomfort or PMDD, because women with PMDD are more likely to develop depression[21] and anxiety disorders later in life, especially panic disorder, phobias, and GAD.[22]

The news isn't all bad: many women who suffer from an anxiety disorder as well as PMDD experience some relief from their anxiety symptoms during the first two weeks after their periods begin. Which leads me to theorize, although I cannot prove it, that a woman's everyday anxiety might also decrease once her period begins.

- **Pregnancy and postpartum.** Pregnancy is notorious for plaguing even the most laid-back gals with worries and wacky dreams that never would have occurred to them were their bodies not humming with hormones and other gestation-friendly biochemicals. We know this because women talk about it, not because there are reams of research to cite. One reason for the paucity of data is that women and scientists alike are loath to engage in any research procedure, however benign-seeming, that might adversely affect a pregnancy. Because of this, almost all research on the prevalence and effects of perinatal anxiety—anxiety occurring shortly before and/or after a birth—has been acquired by asking women to fill out questionnaires. Though this has enabled us to collect information about the symptoms of pregnancy- and postpartum-related anxiety, it has not permitted us to validate the information, as we don't know if the symptoms denote anxiety or physical symptoms associated with the rigors of pregnancy and caring for a newborn. For instance, many of the symptoms on the Beck Anxiety Inventory (a frequently used questionnaire), including sweating, indigestion, facial flushing, difficulty breathing, lightheadedness, and unsteadiness, are common to a normal pregnancy as well as to anxiety.[23] So once again, there is a lot we don't know. Here is a summary of what we do know.

- **Pregnancy seems to ease some symptoms of panic disorder.** I have had more than a few patients tell me that their panic symptoms subsided when they became pregnant. One reason may be that the increase of the hormones prolactin, oxytocin, and cortisol during pregnancy suppresses the stress response sufficiently to blunt anxiety and panicky feelings.[24] Progesterone may also have something to do with it: when it breaks down in the body, by-products are created that have effects similar to benzodiazepines—antianxiety medications—such as clonazepam (marketed under the brand name Klonopin) and diazepam (marketed as Valium).[25] So there may be some truth to the cliché about pregnant women and their air of serenity (until the baby comes, at least).
- **Pregnancy seems to catalyze obsessive-compulsive disorder.** If rising hormone levels during ovulation in-

spire OCD-type behaviors in healthy college students, it should come as no surprise to learn that some women develop OCD for the first time when their hormone levels rise during pregnancy. In a study of 100 pregnant women who did not have an anxiety disorder before they conceived, twenty-five developed obsessive- and compulsive-type symptoms and six developed full-blown OCD while they were pregnant.[26] In cases of new-onset OCD during pregnancy, the emergence of symptoms can be both sudden and intense and may intensify after the baby is born.[27]

- **Women report that their anxiety levels are higher during pregnancy than after their babies are born (with the possible exception of new-onset OCD, as noted above).** In a study of more than eight thousand pregnant women, researchers asked participants to track their anxiety levels while noting how far along they were in their pregnancies. The results showed that more women reported higher anxiety between the eighteenth and thirty-second weeks of their pregnancies—the middle of the second trimester through the middle of the third trimester—than during eight weeks and eight months postpartum.[28] One explanation may be that pregnant women are often anxious about the outcome—Will the birth be painful, difficult, or both? Will the baby be normal? Will they be good mothers?—and are far less so once the birth is over.
- **But postpartum anxiety is common.** Postpartum depression has gotten a lot of press in recent years, but we seldom hear about postpartum anxiety—and we should. Three separate studies found that more than half of women with postpartum anxiety disorders were not depressed and that more women had anxiety disorders after giving birth than had major depres-

sion.[29] In fact, many women—and their partners—experience anxiety after their baby is born.

- **Breast-feeding may diminish postpartum anxiety.** A woman's oxytocin, prolactin, cortisol, and progesterone levels gradually rise during pregnancy and exert anxiety-reducing effects. But the calming effects often diminish rapidly after delivery, when hormone levels fall dramatically (along with, in many cases, a new mother's serenity and high spirits). The good news is that if a woman breast-feeds her infant, her body continues to release oxytocin and prolactin, mitigating the severe drop-off in postpartum hormone levels and extending the suppression of the stress response those hormones provide.[30] Studies show that when a woman breast-feeds she reacts less dramatically to acute stress and that by weaning her infant gradually, she also weans herself gradually from her hormones' calming effects—a much more comfortable return to reality than the cold-turkey approach.

  Sometimes a new mother has trouble breast-feeding and becomes anxious about it: the more anxious she gets, the more trouble she has breast-feeding, until her anxiety about this seeming inability to get it right prompts her to ditch the whole idea and reach for the bottle, so to speak. Ironically, her anxiety about breast-feeding may be the source of the problem: anxiety and stress suppress the release of oxytocin, which is necessary for the release of breast milk. It is quite likely that many women who have trouble breast-feeding would be successful at it if they were aware of—and received help with dissipating—their anxiety.

- **The menopausal transition and beyond.** We hear a lot about forgetfulness and hot flashes and flushes, but not much about the unexpected bouts of anxiety that commonly besiege women as they approach menopause. There is typically a three-to-seven-year transition between a woman's last regular menstrual cycle and her last period. Known as the menopausal transition or perimenopause, this time is characterized by erratic shifts in hormone levels, which may occasionally soar higher than they did earlier in a woman's life. The unpredictability of the shifts makes it difficult to figure out both how much the newfound anxiety is hormone-related and how a woman may expect her everyday anxiety to change once she enters perimenopause. Still, several salient facts have emerged about women's anxiety at midlife:

- **After age fifty, women are no longer twice as likely as men to develop an anxiety disorder.** It seems illogical, but there you are: anxiety is a common symptom of the menopausal transition, yet once women hit midlife, they are less likely to develop an anxiety disorder than when they were younger. Not much research has been done into the effects of menopause on anxiety, so we don't know why this is the case, but the midlife decline of reproductive hormones may very well have something to do with it.
- **Panic symptoms after menopause are fairly common.** A study led by Jordan W. Smoller, M.D., at Massachusetts General Hospital of more than 3,300 postmenopausal women between the ages of fifty and seventy-nine found that nearly 18 percent reported experiencing either a full-blown panic attack or a limited-symptom attack during the six months prior to joining the study. (A full-blown attack would be one comprising the minimum number of symptoms indicating a panic attack, as specified by *DSM-IV.*) Younger participants were more vulnerable to panic symptoms than older ones: the prevalence of full-blown panic attacks was highest among women aged

fifty to fifty-nine. Also, women who had had a full-blown panic attack were likely to have experienced a stressful or painful event during the preceding year.[31] The inference is that as we grow older, it is especially important to be aware of and alleviate as best we can the stresses of both everyday life and extenuating circumstances, as they seem to be associated with the development of panic symptoms (not necessarily panic disorder) later in life.

- **Postmenopausal panic attacks frequently co-occur with other medical problems.** Women who suffer from depression, asthma, emphysema, cardiovascular disease, and migraine headaches are more likely to experience a panic attack after menopause than women without these conditions. The most striking anxiety connection occurs in women who suffer from migraine with aura (when the sufferer perceives flickering lights, spots, and lines in her field of vision): in the Massachusetts General Hospital study, postmenopausal women with a history of this sort of migraine were six times more likely to experience a full-blown panic attack than were women without headaches.[32] Another study (also led by Dr. Smoller at Massachusetts General) found that postmenopausal women who experience panic attacks were three times as likely to suffer a heart attack or stroke within five years of the attack.[33]

Does this mean that postmenopausal women who have a panic attack should fret about developing heart disease? No, it does not. Whereas the study does suggest a connection between anxiety and cardiovascular problems, it is just that—a suggestion—and should be taken with a dose of salt (just a little—too much is unhealthy). When announcing the study's results, Dr. Smoller himself cautioned that the findings were pre-

> liminary and not definitive and admonished those reporting the story to emphasize that the research suggests a possible link and not a direct cause-and-effect relationship between anxiety and heart illness in menopause.

Which brings me to my final point: Don't accept everything that you read as a monolithic truth. Instead, consider the source and weigh the evidence before forming a judgment. In the case of the Massachusetts General studies, they were conducted by teams of established scientists at a world-class research hospital and the results were published in respected medical journals. I would therefore trust the legitimacy of the results, tempered by the admonition of the study's leader, and urge postmenopausal women with panic symptoms not to fret but rather to start paying attention to their heart health (if they haven't already done so) and discuss their cardiovascular condition with their doctors.

As for the quest for truth: I cannot overemphasize the value of cultivating a healthy skepticism when it comes to evaluating what you read, hear, and download. While researching this book, I came across a news story about a study that alleged that women who had abortions were at risk of developing increased anxiety after the procedure. This did not gibe with anything else I had read, so I did a little digging and discovered that the lead author of the study, whose doctorate had been granted by a nonaccredited correspondence school, is a prolife advocate who heads an organization dedicated to abolishing abortion and whose research has been challenged and refuted by several medical experts at major universities. Even so, news outlets printed stories about the research as if it were scientifically sound and free of political motivation. The one I read sounded like a rewrite of a press release from this man's organization, which it very well may have been.

Be wary of what you read: there are promotional pieces out there masquerading as legitimate journalism, and many of us are none the wiser. A press release is not journalism: it is a promotional document that may be announcing legitimate research but is designed to further the agenda, views, and politics of whomever published it. I have neither met this prolife researcher nor studied his data, so I cannot evaluate the merits of his work. But I do know that he lacks the educational credentials and impartiality that characterize those who do legitimate scientific research. I would therefore take his pronouncements with a whopping dose of salt.

part two
THE RELATIONSHIPS

BEFORE WE BEGIN

There is no substitute for the comfort supplied by the utterly taken-for-granted relationship.

—Iris Murdoch[1]

You might say the same of the way we relate to our anxiety: we slip into the most comfortable coping mode as we would an old pair of shoes. Except that, unlike old shoes, comfort is not always a virtue when it comes to managing anxiety. A comfortable coping strategy may be so ingrained that you relax into its rhythm and shuffle through its motions without thinking about what it is you are actually accomplishing, as when you habitually pick up your husband's socks to avoid confronting him, all the while growing more and more annoyed that he leaves his socks around for you to pick up. Yes, the anxiety may abate for a while and permit us to refocus on what we need to think about, but have we really dealt with it? Are our responses to the anxious feelings in proportion to the discomfort they cause? Do they reflect a sober appraisal of the actual threat, or are they a mere habit, as devoid of intention as the hand we run through our hair and the "you know"s and "um"s that slip out of our mouths a hundred times a day?

After many years studying anxiety and working with people who struggle with it, I am convinced that each of us has a relationship with her anxiety—in fact, each of us has a variety of relationships with her different anxieties, much the way we have relationships with different people. As I said earlier, anxiety is something with which each of us is actively engaged, something that we encounter and interact with. I believe that by analyzing the way we relate to our anxiety—indeed, the way*s* we relate to our anxiet*ies*—we can become more aware of the power we have to manage our anxieties and diminish their power over us.

This portion of the book will focus on identifying some of the different kinds of relationships we have with our anxieties and illustrating some of the ways they manifest themselves. I will tell the stories of a variety of women, many of whom were patients (both my own and those of my colleagues) at the Ross Center, and relate their symptoms both as the women described them and as I interpret them. I will then identify the ways I perceived them to be relating to their anxieties and describe some tools and techniques that have been helpful.

My goal is to acquaint you with some relationship archetypes so you may become aware of how you are relating to your anxieties and evaluate whether the relationships are working well for you. To this end, I have come up with four relationship categories: reflexive-impulsive, pervasive-adaptive, primitive-preventive, and imperative-fugitive. These are not the only kinds of relationships; rather, they are categories of my own devising that accommodate most of the anxiety patterns I have observed.

As you read through the relationship chapters, you may recognize yourself and your anxiety patterns in several if not all of them. This is not only normal but desirable; I do not want you to try and fit yourself into any one category. In fact, I urge you to resist it. This would defeat the purpose of the work by oversimplifying the nature of anxiety and our responses to it. Keep your mind open and refrain from labeling yourself as one type or another; in fact, most people have a variety of anxiety relationships and will find each category familiar in some way. If this isn't the case with you, that's fine, too; some women have a narrower coping repertoire and will see themselves as operating in only one or two categories. The important thing is to be open and consider aspects of yourself you may not have perceived before. Just as I asked you to fill out all the anxiety questionnaires at the end of Chapter 2, so I ask you to read all the relationship chapters in this section of the book. Even if it turns out that, say, you have a mostly imperative-fugitive relationship with your anxiety—in other words, you usually try to manage it by running from it and avoiding anxiety-provoking situations—you may still discover that you have a touch of pervasive-adaptive lurking within you and have crafted some aspects of your life to constructively accommodate and even capitalize on your anxiety. Just glimpsing this unexpected aspect of yourself can reveal a source of strength you didn't know you had and encourage you to confront and perhaps even control some of the anxieties you had been running from.

I want you to see yourself with clear, new eyes, to take the Pandora's box in which you have stashed your anxieties and think outside of it. I want you to develop an awareness of the relationships you have with your anxieties so you can take charge of them and make them serve rather than manipulate you.

four

THE REFLEXIVE-IMPULSIVE RELATIONSHIP

Reflexive: without conscious thought

Impulsive: acting without forethought

The essence of the reflexive-impulsive relationship is its lack of forethought: when you relate to anxiety in this way, you do things to relieve it in the moment without evaluating their usefulness or weighing the consequences of your actions. This does not necessarily mean that what you are doing is harmful, but it does mean that you are operating in *que será, será* mode—that is, *I'll do what works right here, right now, and as for the future—whatever will be, will be.*

By calling the relationship reflexive, I mean to invoke the body's involuntary, predictable response when it is stimulated in a certain way, as when a doctor taps your knee with a little rubber hammer and your foot flies up as if it had received an electric shock. The response seems oddly incongruous to the stimulus, yet there it is: a gentle knock on the knee produces an automatic reaction whose purpose is as obscure as it is robust. So it is with people who relate this way to their anxiety: their responses to anxiety tend to be as involuntary and as robust as the effectiveness and consequences of these responses are unexamined.

The impulsive aspect of this relationship lies in the spontaneous decisions we make and actions we take to quell the anxiousness. It takes many forms: one woman may consume an entire layer cake, whereas another may charge a thousand dollars' worth of merchandise she can't afford, while yet another may blurt out an ill-advised dinner party invitation before she realizes that her action was an unwitting attempt to relieve anxiety. You know the feeling: the pressure builds up inside you like steam in a kettle, and something's got to give. So you eat or you spend or you blurt, and for a few seconds the pressure is eased—but not for long: pretty soon the anxiety starts building anew and the reflex kicks in until you again do something impulsive to relieve the tension.

I want to emphasize that such impulsive actions may not be destructive in themselves (although eating an entire layer cake probably is); what makes them warrant scrutiny is not their inherent unsuitability but their side effects and ramifications.

I also want to emphasize that having a reflexive-impulsive relationship with your anxiety doesn't mean you are utterly oblivious to the consequences of your actions (although we all are, from time to time); it means there are things you automatically do—actions you take, words you use, behaviors you manifest—to relieve the mounting sensation of anxiety. The things you do may be helpful, they may be detrimental, or they may be neither; they will in fact differ in their effects depending on the situation you are using them to address. The defining characteristic of this anxiety relationship is not the efficacy of the responses it catalyzes but its unplanned, fix-it-quick quality. The responses may work well for a person or they may not work so well, as when they cause a person's anxiety to manifest in a different way.

TERESA: "I'M WAY TOO STRESSED TO DO YOGA"

I was eagerly anticipating the flight to London as I buckled myself into my seat. As stressful as air travel can be since 9/11, I still look forward to transatlantic flights because they offer me a seven-hour stretch when I don't have to talk on the phone or respond to emails: it's just me, reading I need to catch up on, and a nice, solitary snooze through the night. I seldom if ever converse with my seatmate because once that little pillow is tucked behind my head and a blanket around my knees, there isn't much that can keep me from going into hermit mode.

Except chocolate. Chocolate is one thing for which I make an exception. And from the look of it, that's exactly what my seatmate was dangling in front of me.

"Pardon me, but would you care for a truffle?"

Boy, would I ever. I nodded and was soon enjoying one of the most delectable dark chocolate confections I had ever tasted, an opinion I shared with my benefactor.

"I'm glad to hear you say that," she said. "I was a little concerned they might taste too dark, if you know what I mean. But so far, everyone who's tried them has loved them."

Her name was Teresa, and she was the head of product development for a high-end chocolatier (now, how do you get a job like *that*?). She was bound for Geneva and a meeting on the newly discovered cardiovascular benefits of dark chocolate (this was a few years ago) and how to convince the health-conscious American public that bonbon consumption was actually good for their hearts. We chatted about the studies showing that cocoa and chocolate seemed to lower blood pressure and prevent fatty substances from clogging blood vessels, all the while enhancing our heart health, one truffle at a time. She asked what I did for a living, and I told her I was heading to an anxiety conference in London, after which I begged her pardon and said I wanted to try to sleep until we got there.

"I hope you don't mind if I keep my light on," she said, "but I'm going to be up the whole time."

"That's okay," I said, "I know a lot of people who have trouble sleeping on planes."

"It's not just planes; I can't sleep anywhere. But I get a lot of work done between midnight and three, especially over the Atlantic. I just hope I can stay awake tomorrow. But"—she stopped and held her hands up, palms toward me—"if I start telling you my story now, you won't get any sleep either. Maybe I could come in and talk to you when we're back in D.C."

About six weeks later she was in my office. Teresa was forty-five, and now that we were in daylight I could see she looked older. There were purplish half circles under her eyes, and every so often she would lower her eyelids and take a deep breath as if to rouse herself.

"My insomnia got really bad last year," she said. "My daughter, Kristyn, was a freshman at Arizona State, and it wasn't working out. The school was too big, she was too far away, the friend she had gone there to be with was spending all her time with her boyfriend; she was miserable. She called every night, and we'd be on the phone forever, her crying and blaming me for encouraging her to go there, me telling her that things would get better and she should stick it out. By the time we'd hang up, it would be past midnight and then it would take me at least an hour to calm down. So I'd doze off at one or two in the morning, and then I'd have to be up again at six to go to work.

"Then, in the midst of all this, my father was diagnosed with cancer. My mother's gone and he lives alone, so I took on his medical care, dealing with doctors, arranging the surgery, his convalescence, everything. Between dealing with Kristyn and staying up till all hours surfing the Web for cancer information, I was down to two, maybe three hours of sleep a night. When I was lucky."

"You're an only child?"

"No, I have two brothers. But I'm older, so they figure it's my job to handle everything and they're hassling me over the phone every night. So I'd hang up with Nick and Vince would call, and I'd hang up with him and Kristyn would call, and"—she took a deep breath—"you get the idea."

I did. I learned more: Teresa had married Ed, her college boyfriend, after graduation; he took an editing job and she worked while going for an MBA at night. After graduation Teresa landed a job with a gourmet food importer; the starting salary was good, the benefits were great, and the couple decided to have a baby. Kristyn was born four years into the marriage; not long afterward, Ed quit his job and started writing freelance from home. But he soon found he couldn't meet deadlines while caring for an infant and Kristyn was placed in full-time day care. As Teresa's income grew, she and Ed began to argue about money: Teresa thought Ed should take a full-time publishing position—Kristyn was in day care, after all—and contribute more to the family's upkeep. But Ed demurred; the corporate world was not for him, he said, and he was devoting quality time to Kristyn and the family while Teresa was out growing her career. The marriage lasted fourteen years; Kristyn was ten when Teresa and Ed divorced, after which Kristyn shuttled between them in a joint custody arrangement.

"That's when the stress really kicked in," Teresa said. "Kristyn would come home after spending time with Ed, and I'd hear about all this stuff they'd do together—he'd go and have lunch with her at school or chaperone class trips—daytime stuff that I couldn't do because of my job. So I started telecommuting two days a week, which was great for having chicken nuggets in the school cafeteria but not for my career. I began to lose ground, and I couldn't afford that—who was going to pay for Kristyn's college?—so I went back five days a week."

"What was Kristyn's reaction?"

"She became clingy, which was new for her. She began to worry when I traveled and actually turned down a chance to go to New York with her class because she didn't want to be that far away from her father and me, even for a weekend. Which is why I thought it was good when she decided to go to school in Arizona: I was dying to have her closer but was pleased she was asserting her independence."

Then came some relief: Teresa's father went into remission and back to his own house; Kristyn joined the staff of the student newspaper and Arizona State became the greatest school on the planet; and Teresa was getting between five and six hours of sleep a night—a bonanza for her.

But now Teresa's insomnia had returned. She had been made a vice president and gotten a raise—a fine development—but had been promoted over a more senior colleague who now reported to her and was making no secret of his discontent. She was also traveling more often. Overseas travel disrupts the sleep patterns of even loglike slumberers, and for Teresa the disruption was profound. With meetings in Europe every six to eight weeks, her internal clock barely had time to adjust before it was jarred out of whack again. As weary as she felt at night, she would no sooner close her eyes than she was besieged by visions of the tasks she had left undone, calls she had yet to make, and conflicts she had left unresolved. She forced herself out of bed in the morning through sheer willpower but found it harder and harder to focus at work and stay awake at meetings. It was taking her more and more time to accomplish less and less, and she had begun to fret about keeping up at work, which compounded her anxiety and made it even harder to sleep.

First Impressions

Teresa's inability to relax was directly tied to her feeling overwhelmed by situations she felt responsible for managing, fixing, and healing: her father's illness, her brothers' discontent, her daughter's neediness, and, not least, conflicts and crises at work. Like many women (and eldest children), Teresa felt it was her job to promote the happiness and well-being of the people around her, even when those people were adults and ought to have been doing it for themselves.

I see this over and over again: women who suffer from relentless, low- to midlevel anxiety that allows them to perform all their daily functions except the one that is perhaps most important to their overall well-being: detaching from their daily obligations sufficiently to unwind and turn their minds to something else. These women are typically competent, thorough, and organized and thrive on doing several things at once; they are highly efficient at work, and their families run like well-oiled machines. But they find they cannot relax—neither at the end of the day, nor, in many cases, on weekends or on vacation—enough to focus on anything besides their chores without drinking a glass of wine, taking a sleeping pill, or engaging in bouts of nervous eating and impulsive activity that comfort them in a vague but ultimately unsatisfying way. The results, which often include weight gain, fatigue, body tightness, headaches, muscle pain, back spasms, diminished ability to concentrate, and chronic inability to fall asleep and/or stay asleep, can wreak havoc with a woman's relationships, career, and overall health, especially over time.

Determining the Anxiety Relationship

To learn how Teresa related to her anxiety, I needed to ask her how she perceived both her symptoms and her responses to those symptoms, which I did at our next session.

"The symptoms change a lot, depending on what's going on in my life," she said. "When Kristyn was unhappy at school, all I'd need to do was hear her voice on the phone and my head would start pounding. During the fights with my brothers, I'd feel as if my guts were on fire. Sometimes I get so worked up I feel like I'm going to explode."

"What do you do then?"

"Different things. I might take a pill for a headache, or when I'm on the phone with my brother, I start pacing up and down the stairs. Once I hang up, I'll maybe turn on the TV, do some laundry, grab something to eat, a piece of cake or something, but nothing really works. It still takes me at least an hour to calm down. Sometimes I wake up in the morning and I'm still stressed from the night before."

"Are you getting any exercise?"

"Not for a while; I just don't have the time to go to the gym."

"How about something you could do at home, like yoga?"

"Yoga? I'm way too stressed to do yoga."

Saying you're too stressed to do yoga is tantamount to saying you're too out of shape to go to the gym. Teresa definitely had a sense of humor.

"Tell me about your sleep patterns. Is it that you can't fall asleep, or do you fall asleep and wake up?"

"It's hard for me to fall asleep at all unless I stay up until I collapse. If I turn out the light just because it's getting late, I can lie awake for hours."

"What do you do when that happens?"

"Sometimes I just toss and turn until I conk out. But that sometimes doesn't happen until three in the morning and then I'm a wreck the next day. So then I might turn on the TV or go to the kitchen and get something to snack on. Last week I got up and started painting the powder room—I'm doing this sponge-on glaze in several rooms in the house. Or I might get my laptop and work until I pass out."

"How often does this happen?"

"Not too often; maybe two or three times a week"—two or three sleepless nights a week was *not too often*? I marveled that this woman was even able to sit up in a chair—"but on the nights when I do fall asleep quickly, I wake up in the middle of the night at two or three or four, and every time I look at the clock I get more and more anxious about how late it is and how little sleep I'm going to get. And pretty soon my heart is thumping and I can forget about sleeping, so I get up and onto the computer until it's time to leave for work."

"What about alcohol?"

"Never touch the stuff. My mother was an alcoholic, and I saw what drinking did to her."

"Or drugs?"

"Nothing there either, except maybe ibuprofen for a headache."

"What time do you usually go to bed?"

"No set time; I go to bed when I think I might be able to fall asleep."

"Can you describe a typical evening?"

"There's nothing typical about my evenings. It's just me, so there's no need for a routine."

I smiled. "Actually, having a routine can be helpful. But what I meant was, what time do you get home? When do you have dinner, and what do you usually eat?"

"Some nights I work late and eat some cheese and crackers when I get home; other nights I'll pop a frozen dinner in the microwave. Sometimes I go out with friends, and then what I eat depends on where we go."

"What else do you do at night?"

"It depends on how I'm feeling. I might do some work on the house—I've got three rooms started so far—or I'll go on the computer, do some online shopping, deal with my email. Mostly I'll just try to catch up on work."

"Where do you do the work?"

"If I'm eating, I'll work at the kitchen table, and sometimes I work in bed. I know they say you shouldn't do that, but I never finish at the office, and I do find it relaxing to know I'm catching up."

"Do you watch TV in bed?"

"Well, I might pop in a DVD or put on one of those home shopping shows while I'm working. I also catch up on my emails when I can't sleep."

"Work emails?"

"No, personal stuff. Nick and Vince are happy to let me handle everything—unless, of course, I do something they don't like. Like when I put Dad in assisted living to convalesce near me, and all of a sudden they're very involved: Why does he have to be in Washington? Why can't he be near them, where it's cheaper?—as if either of them would ever visit him. Not only do I have to take care of everything, they give me a hard time about it—"

"Teresa, stop for a moment. What are you feeling right now?"

She looked startled. "What am I feeling?"

"Yes—right now: What are you feeling?"

"I'm ticked off, that's what I'm feeling. I do everything for my father; I do everything for everybody! Nobody can do anything for themselves unless I've done the research or made the phone call or written the letter—well, hello. I know what you're thinking."

"And what is that?"

"You're thinking that it's pretty obvious why I can't sleep at night. It's because I get myself all worked up when I should be winding down." Touché.

"How do you prepare for bed?"

"I take off my clothes, put them away, take off my makeup, wash my face, brush my teeth—you know, the usual."

"Do you lay out your clothes for the next day?"

"No, but I probably should because sometimes when I can't sleep I start obsessing about what I should wear the next day and wondering what the weather's going to be like, and then I really can't fall asleep."

"You mentioned a clock. Tell me about the arrangement of things in your room."

"There's a chest of drawers, dresser, TV, and a chair. Piles of books, magazines, and a stack of printouts from work that I brought home to read and never brought back. There's a night table with a digital clock, books, receipts, hand cream, magazines, the newspaper—a real mess. Oh, and the mail—sometimes when I can't sleep, I'll get a snack and go through the mail."

Anxiety Disorder, Sleep Disorder, or Everyday Anxiety?

When I first met Teresa, I thought she might have generalized anxiety disorder: muscle tension, fatigue, difficulty sleeping, and gastrointestinal discomfort are common GAD symptoms, and Teresa had them all. But the more I learned about Teresa, the more I felt that although she had some GAD symptoms, she did not have GAD. People with GAD tend to suffer from persistent, excessive, and unrealistic worry about everyday things, but Teresa's worries, however persistent, were neither excessive nor unrealistic when you looked at the circumstances of her life. Teresa's anxieties were the result of everyday stresses that many of us eventually face—an elderly, ailing parent, a child's insecurity, a demanding career. But unlike some of us, Teresa was shouldering these burdens alone: she lived alone, was not close enough to anyone who might lend emotional support, and, at forty-five, was still playing the in-charge, big-sister role opposite her brothers. She was also approaching middle age and could be in the early stages of perimenopause, which might have increased her vulnerability to anxiety and sleep disruptions.

Nor did I think Teresa had a sleep disorder; had I thought that likely, I would have referred her to a clinic that specialized in diagnosing and treating such ailments. Based on my observations of and conversations with Teresa, I believed her problem was rooted in anxiety even though its dominant manifestation was insomnia. I set about treating her as I would an anxiety patient.

The first step was to help Teresa see how chaotic her prebedtime hours were. Whereas Teresa was self-aware when it came to the small picture—she could tell me, for example, that she knew she shouldn't be working in bed or habitually dozing off with the television on—she was not seeing the bigger, broader patterns of impulsive behaviors that were quelling her anxiety in the moment but carving an inner landscape in which rest and renewal were impossible. To increase Teresa's awareness of her behaviors, I gave her two sets of forms to fill out before her next session: a personal habits diary, and a sleep diary.

Personal Habits Diary

I designed this form to help Teresa do two things: identify the anxiety-related feelings that beset her at night and become aware of the reflexive and impulsive ways she typically responded to the anxiety. The form required her to jot down information that she might otherwise consider insignificant, such as what time she came home from work, what time she ate dinner, and what she ate; if and when she exercised each day and what exercise she did; what time she woke up in the morning and what time she got into bed; what she did once she was in bed (whom she spoke to, emailed, or wrote to); what websites she was visiting; and what books, publications, or work-related material she was reading. In addition, she was to write down any and all anxious thoughts that intruded into her mind during the hours leading up to her bedtime (such as it was), noting where she was, what she was doing, and whom she was with (or talking to on the phone or emailing) when the intrusive thoughts occurred.

"But I can tell you everything right now," Teresa said. "It's pretty much the same thing every night."

That's where she was wrong: if it really were the same thing every night, she would have a routine, and if she had a routine, she would probably be sleeping better. I was firm: Teresa was to complete the personal habits diary; moreover, she was to be as precise as possible, not merely writing "I'm worried about Dad" but identifying specific fears, such as "I'm anxious that Dad's cancer will return and he won't tell me about the symptoms until it's too late." The more specific she was about what was triggering her anxiety, the more effectively she could apply a safety to the trigger and prevent the anxiety from going off.

Keeping a detailed record of your thoughts and behaviors isn't difficult, but it does require both intention and attention, which was exactly what Teresa needed to work on. Once you write something down, it becomes more real. I wanted Teresa to see a week's worth of reality in writing. Mentioning scraps of it from memory would not do the trick, but I had a hunch that writing it all down would. (I designed the personal habits diary for Teresa based on what I knew her problems to be—which were, as it happens, typical of many people who have trouble sleeping. I have reproduced a blank copy of the two-sided form on pages 96–97 and invite you to photocopy and use it if you think it might be helpful to you.)

Sleep Diary

The second part of Teresa's assignment was to keep a record of her sleeping habits over the next seven days. Keeping a sleep diary means you write down all the minutiae that may possibly affect if, how, and how well you sleep: the time you got into bed and the time you dragged yourself out of it; the time you fell asleep (or imagine you did); the times you woke up during the night; the total number of hours (or minutes, on a really bad night) you think you slept; what, if anything, disturbed your sleep; and how much caffeine you ingested, exercise you completed, food you ate, medications you took, and activities you did before getting into bed and trying to sleep. Several of the categories overlapped those of the personal habits diary, but no matter: I wanted Teresa to complete both forms in full. (The sleep diary did not originate with me; the excerpt that follows is adapted from one created by the National Sleep Foundation, whose version can be found at its website, www.sleepfoundation.org, along with information on the benefits of sleep and consequences of not getting enough of it. More contact information for the National Sleep Foundation appears on page 244.)

PERSONAL HABITS DIARY (PAGE 1)

Day and Date:	*I woke up today at:*	*I got out of bed today at:*	*I ate dinner at:*	*What I ate for dinner:*	*Exercise I did today:*	*Alcohol, caffeine, drugs I used:*	*Bedtime preparations and routine:*

PERSONAL HABITS DIARY (PAGE 2)

Day and Date:	*TV, DVDs, other media I watched before bed:*	*After-dinner snack(s) I ate and time(s):*	*Nature of nighttime phone calls, emails, conversations, etc.:*	*Time I turned off the light:*	*Intrusive thoughts:*	*What I did when I couldn't sleep:*

SLEEP DIARY: DATE ___________

COMPLETE IN THE MORNING

I got into bed last night at:	*I got out of bed today at:*	*Last night, I fell asleep in:*	*I woke up during the night:*
_______ P.M./A.M.	_______ A.M./P.M.	_____ minutes	# of times _____ # of minutes _____

When I woke up for the day, I felt:	*Last night I slept a total of:*	*My sleep was disturbed by (list any mental, physical, and/or environmental factors):*
❑ refreshed ❑ somewhat refreshed ❑ fatigued	_____ hours	______________________ ______________________ ______________________

COMPLETE AT THE END OF THE DAY

I consumed caffeinated drinks in the:	*I exercised at least 20 minutes in the:*	*Approximately 2–3 hours before going to bed, I consumed:*
❑ morning ❑ afternoon ❑ evening ❑ not applicable	❑ morning ❑ afternoon ❑ evening ❑ not applicable	❑ alcohol ❑ a heavy meal ❑ not applicable

Medication(s) I took today:	*About 1 hour before getting into bed, I did the following activities:*
______________________ ______________________ ______________________	______________________ ______________________

On a scale of 0 to 4, with 0 being "falling asleep" and 4 being "wide awake," write down the number that best represents how sleepy you felt (or feel) during the time frames below:

_____	_____	_____	_____
Morning (6 A.M.–12 P.M.)	*Afternoon (12 P.M.–6 P.M.)*	*Evening (6 P.M.–12 A.M.)*	*Night (12 A.M.–6 A.M.)*

Adapted and reprinted with permission of the National Sleep Foundation.

A week later, Teresa strode into my office.

"I didn't think I needed to do this personal habits thing, but, boy, was it an eye-opener."

It wasn't a complete eye-opener for me, as I could have guessed the gist of many of her responses. Here's a summary of the first-week entries in Teresa's personal habits diary:

Waking and getting-out-of-bed times: 6:00 A.M. Monday through Friday. Slept until 11:30 on Saturday and noon on Sunday.

Dinner time: Different every night: sometimes 7:30; one night, 11:30.

What I ate for dinner: Monday, frozen low-fat entrée; Tuesday, barbecued ribs; Wednesday, Chinese takeout; Thursday, out late with friends, ate a steak, took longer than usual to fall asleep; Friday, salad at 8:00, woke up hungry at 3:00, raided refrigerator.

Exercise: 15 sit-ups on Saturday.

Caffeine, alcohol, drugs: No alcohol. Ibuprofen on Wednesday and Friday nights for headache. Drank two cups of coffee in morning but never past 10:00 A.M.

Bedtime preparations and routine: Some nights in bed at 10:00, others, not till 1:00. Removed makeup some nights but not always; nothing else in particular.

TV, movies, other media I watched before bed: Put in a movie two nights; watched late-night talk shows and shopping channels until 1:30 two nights.

After-dinner snacks I ate and time(s): Tuesday, bowl of cold cereal, 10:00; Wednesday, reheated pasta and sauce, 11:00; Friday, chocolate milk shake at drive-thru, midnight.

Nature of nighttime phone calls, emails, etc.: Logged on to Internet Monday at 11:45 after Dad's call about dizziness, logged off at 1:25; took phone calls past 10:30 from Nick and Vince, got emails afterward—arrrgh!—couldn't fall asleep until past 2:00 several nights. On phone 11:30 to 1:00 A.M. with Kristyn Saturday while she cried about Andrew.

Time I turned off the light: Not sure. Between 1:00 and 2:00 several times; other nights, typically after midnight.

Intrusive thoughts: Kristyn wouldn't have these romantic problems if I hadn't gotten divorced; Dad didn't tell me he was dizzy for several days—what else is he hiding? Something bad's going to happen to him because he doesn't tell me what's going on; Vince and Nick will write me off once Dad is gone; what if that weasel Dilbert penalizes me for taking all those personal days last month?

What I did when I couldn't sleep: Watched QVC, ordered carpet shampooer and leather repair kit; started new Patricia Cornwell; Thursday, started reorganizing closet at 11:00, woke up at 4:00 A.M. in a pile of old skirts.

Now I had enough to go on.

Teresa's Anxiety Relationship: Reflexive-Impulsive

Teresa's verbal description of her symptoms made me guess that she had a reflexive-impulsive relationship with her anxiety; her diaries convinced me. Everything pointed to it: random dinner times, hit-or-miss meals and snacking, haphazard sleep hygiene—behaviors and surroundings that are not conducive to a good night's sleep—and varying bedtimes, stress-inducing bedtime activities, and scattershot behaviors when she could not sleep. She was aware that she needed to change the way she was managing her anxiety. But when the anxiety actually hit, she would revert to acting without thinking, doing this and that in slapdash attempts to calm herself enough to fall sleep.

What Teresa had to do—and what anyone with this anxiety relationship has to do—was become aware of her anxiety *before* she acted on it so she could change her mindless responses to mindful ones. Like other people with insomnia, Teresa would often try to solve problems at night and start her mind racing when she should have been calming down. To help Teresa break this cycle, she needed to improve her sleep hygiene, which would involve breaking some ingrained habits, creating some new ones, and adjusting the environment.

Treatment Plan

- **Improve your sleep hygiene and overall health.** Teresa and I sat down and went over her diary entries. Because so many of her behaviors were not conducive to good health, we agreed that it made sense for her to work on two things: improving her health-related behaviors and deactivating her individual insomnia triggers. What follows is a rundown of new behaviors Teresa and I designed to transform her mindless responses into mindful ones (which might be useful to anyone, whether or not she has sleeping difficulties). Together we were able to identify proactive, health-promoting behaviors that Teresa could incorporate into her daily routine to replace the impulsive behaviors that were simply a response to her anxiety.
- **New health-promoting behaviors**
    - **Dinnertime.** Make a serious effort to eat dinner at about the same time every night, preferably between

7:00 and 9:00 P.M. Try to complete the meal at least three hours before bedtime.

- **Dinner menu.** Plan ahead so you can easily prepare a nutritious, well-balanced dinner. A healthy diet emphasizes fruits, vegetables, whole grains, and fat-free or low-fat milk and milk products. It also includes lean meats, poultry, fish, beans, eggs, and nuts and is low in saturated fats, trans fats, cholesterol, salt (sodium), and added sugars. With this in mind, keep salad fixings, frozen vegetables, fish, chicken breasts, and soy products on hand, so even if there isn't much time to cook, you can throw together a salad and stir-fry easily and quickly. A good way to be sure your meal is balanced is to think about how the dinner plate will look. Vegetables and salads should take up about half the plate; one quarter of the plate should be occupied by lean protein such as fish, soy products, or lean meat, beans, or skinless chicken; and the last quarter should be composed of whole grains such as brown rice, whole-wheat pasta, bulgur wheat, or buckwheat groats. Incorporate some healthy fat, such as olive or canola oil, by using it for sautéing or as salad dressing; a few chunks of avocado or a handful of nuts (unsalted ones, either raw or dry-roasted, are healthiest, of course) also contain natural, healthful fat. And if you haven't had fruit or fat-free or low-fat milk products earlier in the day, be sure to include those as well, perhaps for dessert. Pay particular attention to avoiding spicy or fatty foods, which can cause gas and heartburn.
- **Have a light snack before bed.** It is important that you select carefully what you eat immediately prior to going to bed. Some foods may actually help bring on sleep as they contain tryptophan, an amino acid that the body converts to serotonin. A glass of warm low-

fat milk is a good source of tryptophan (add a dash of nutmeg for flavor, if you wish), as are cottage cheese, peanut butter, yogurt, banana, sesame seeds, nuts, and poultry (skinless, white-meat chicken or turkey with a slice of whole-wheat bread or toast is an ideal bed-time snack). Avoid foods that contain caffeine, such as chocolate, caffeinated coffee and tea, and certain soft drinks, especially colas. Also, resist the temptation to eat anything containing a large amount of sugar (often appearing in the form of high-fructose corn syrup). Snacking on something high in sugar can lead to blood sugar fluctuations that may keep you awake.

- **Exercise.** Incorporate physical exercise into your daily routine, choosing activities that you enjoy and are readily available. Do not, for example, vow to swim after work four times a week if the nearest pool is ten miles in the opposite direction from your house; you will soon weary of the commute and grow landlocked. A good goal is to do a minimum of thirty minutes of aerobic exercise at least four times a week. Keep yourself motivated by trying different activities on different days, perhaps alternating between bicycling and taking a spin class, taking a step aerobics or dance class, taking long, vigorous walks or runs with a friend or colleague, or going to a martial arts class. What is most important is to be physically active most days of the week and to make exercise part of your daily routine.

  In addition to formal exercise activities, take advantage of everyday opportunities to get your heart pumping. These could include taking the stairs rather than an elevator or escalator, walking briskly to and from the parking lot, subway station, or bus stop, or taking several ten-minute breaks during the day to walk around the block a few times. These sound simple and obvious, but their salutary effects add up.

Keep a pair of serviceable walking or running shoes and some comfortable clothes in your office or car so if there's an opportunity for some exercise during the day, you can grab it.

Whereas doing half an hour of aerobic exercise early in the day can help you fall asleep and stay asleep at night, doing it in the evening could have the opposite effect. Since exercise stimulates the body, doing aerobic exercise close to bedtime can make falling asleep difficult, even for people who don't have sleep problems. It is best to avoid aerobic activity within three or four hours of going to bed (except for sex, a time-honored anxiety buster).

- **Waking time.** Wake up on weekends at a set time and not too late. Sleeping very late on weekends when you have to wake up early during the week can wreak havoc with your body clock.
- **Bedroom environment.** Remove distractions. Take steps to make the bedroom conducive to sleep: more serene and less stimulating.
    - **Neaten up the room.** Books and periodicals may remain as long as they're orderly, but work-related reading material must go. Tidy up the night table. Remove clutter (a visually chaotic environment is not psychologically restful); go through the mail elsewhere, not in the bedroom, and do it well before bedtime so that you don't start worrying about unpaid bills.
    - **Pivot your alarm clock so it faces away from the bed or cover it so the display is not visible** (do this right before turning out the light). When you can't sleep or wake up in the middle of the night, seeing the time can ramp up your anxiety. It's counterproductive to make yourself aware of every passing second when you're trying to relax.

  - **Keep work out of the bedroom**—no laptop, no files, no reading, no nothing. Leave your briefcase and all work-related materials in another part of the house. This will enforce an image of the bedroom as a place dedicated to the pursuit of sleep (and the expression of intimacy).
  - **Remove the TV.** (See "TV, movies, and other media," below.)
- **Bedtime preparations and routine.** Establish a consistent presleep routine and stick to it. Undress and hang up your clothes, remove your makeup and perform your beauty rituals, brush your teeth, and turn out the light at the same time each night; make sure your alarm is set for the same time each morning. Some other suggestions:
  - **Lay out the next day's outfit.** This won't work for everyone; there are some women who prefer to wake up and see what they feel like wearing rather than decide the night before. Even if you're one of them, making decisions in advance about what you'll be wearing may save you just enough mental activity to calm you a bit more before bed. It's worth a try.
  - **Keep the bedroom temperature on the cool side.** Most people sleep more soundly in a cool room. Also, if a woman is in perimenopause, she may have hot flushes while she sleeps (night sweats), which may wake her up. Keeping the bedroom cooler won't stop the nighttime flushes, but it won't make them feel any more intense than they already do, whereas a warm bedroom might.
  - **Darken the room as bedtime approaches.** Lower the blinds, close the curtains or drapes; turn off the overhead light in favor of a bedside lamp (and consider using a lower-wattage bulb in the lamp).
  - **Reading is okay, but nothing work-related.** Magazines and books are okay as long as they don't rile you

up. *Sheep!* magazine is probably fine; *The Silence of the Lambs* is definitely not.

- **Caffeine, alcohol, drugs.** Some coffee in the morning is fine but not past noon lest the caffeine remain in your system and inhibit sleep at night. Some people can drink caffeinated coffee after dinner and fall asleep with no problem, but for someone with insomnia, limiting caffeine intake to the morning is a sound preventive measure. (I didn't bring up alcohol or drug use with Teresa because she said she didn't use any, beyond an occasional ibuprofen. Had drugs and/or alcohol been contributing to Teresa's problem, I would have addressed them.)
- **TV, movies, and other media (including computers).** Remove the TV from the room—no watching TV in the bedroom, period. In addition to the psychological effect of being bombarded by images close to bedtime, there is also a biological effect: studies are showing that the blue light emitted by computer and television screens may trick the body into thinking it's morning and sending signals to wake up.[1] (To counteract this effect, some therapists prescribe yellow-tinted goggles that cancel out blue light for people who have to work late in front of a computer monitor.) You could argue that watching TV in the boudoir is not a problem if it's daytime and you're not trying to sleep, and I'd argue back that that would be fine if you weren't suffering from insomnia. If you are and part of your pattern is to have the TV on for either part of the evening or all night long, it's best to remove the monitor (and the temptation to watch it) from the bedroom altogether.
- **Snacking before bed.** Eat a healthy snack in the kitchen before getting into bed. Again, it should be something light and healthy, such as fruit or a slice of turkey.
- **Nature of nighttime phone calls, emails, etc.** Set boundaries. Dealing with emotionally draining personal issues at

night is an ingrained pattern that might take a while to change. Some ways to start:

- **Establish a cutoff time for phone calls and emails.** Tell family members (and friends, if that's who is calling and emailing you) that you will not be answering the phone or checking emails past a certain time—say, nine o'clock—and ask that they not contact you unless the matter is urgent. Of course, there will be times when you do have to take late-evening calls, but setting a general nine o'clock deadline will discourage both casual chitchat calls as well as those that are important but can wait until the next day.
- **Do not check your email past a certain time.** This takes discipline but is absolutely worth it: there's nothing like opening a high-impact, stress-inducing email late at night to wreck your sleeping prospects.
- **Make it a habit to check your caller ID** to see who's phoning before picking up, especially if the phone rings later than you would like to talk. This also takes discipline, especially if you're the kind of person who leaps up to answer the phone whenever it rings. But if you can refrain from answering after a certain time, late-calling friends and family members will eventually get the idea.

- **Intrusive thoughts.** Keep a notepad and pen on your night table. If you find yourself fretting while trying to fall asleep, or if you wake up in the middle of night worried about something, jot it down on the pad and tell yourself you will deal with it in the morning. This technique works by conceptualizing anxious thoughts as concrete commodities—intangible yet actual things—that you can remove from your consciousness by giving them someplace to go (onto the notepad) and over which you can exercise a satisfying degree of control. By jotting down your bothersome thoughts, they symbolically exit your mind, freeing it to tread more tranquil ground.

- **What to do when you can't sleep:**
    - **Try a relaxation exercise, such as a self-guided visualization.** Picture yourself walking along a deserted beach and listening to the rhythmic breaking of the waves; or sitting on a mountaintop, serenaded by birds; or being somewhere else that makes you feel tranquil. Note what colors you see, sounds you hear, and odors you smell. By distancing yourself from anxiety-provoking thoughts and focusing on repetitive, lulling images or activities (hence the wisdom of counting sheep), you will help your brain shut down and move into sleep mode.
    - **If thirty minutes have passed and you are still lying there awake,** get out of bed, go into another room, and do something relaxing until you feel sleepy: read a book or magazine, knit, crochet, or cross-stitch; practice the guitar; write in your journal. Don't turn on the TV, though, as you are likely to get sucked into something that will either keep you up for hours or inundate you with images that are not conducive to sleep. Changing your environment helps break the anxious thoughts that spiral when you're lying in bed awake.

I saw Teresa weekly for the next month and a half and was heartened by her progress: rather than try to change everything at once, she made small, significant changes and found that worked well for her (as it does for most people). She was proudest of joining a local running club that met at 7:30 A.M. twice a week and of the fact that, other than one time when she was out of the country, she hadn't missed a single run. She began going to the market over the weekend and stocking up on good foods, which enabled her to have better control over her evening eating habits during the week. And she did a bedroom makeover: now referring to the bedroom as her "sleep sanctuary," Teresa relocated the television to another room, decluttered her night table, and cleared the space of distractions (especially papers from work). She also told her daughter and brothers about her new anti-insomnia regimen and enlisted their support by asking them to phone her no later than nine at night unless it was an emergency. She said they had all agreed.

RENÉE: "I'M SORRY, BUT I CAN'T RELATE TO ALL THIS ANXIETY STUFF. I'M JUST NOT AN ANXIOUS PERSON"

Walk up to any woman and ask if anxiety figures into her day-to-day life, and she's likely to say yes, it sure does. Any woman, that is, except Renée.

We at the Ross Center would never have met Renée were it not for her son, whose pediatrician referred him to a therapist on my staff after noting the teenager's reddened, raw-looking fingers and his reluctance to shake the doctor's hand after the appointment. A lanky fifteen-year-old whose hair hung nearly to his shoulders, Adam said his fear of germs and need to scrub his hands throughout the day had gotten a lot worse starting about six months earlier. As it happened, that was when his mother had announced her plans to marry a widower with two daughters, all three of whom she had recently invited to move in with her and Adam without consulting her son.

"It was, like, they were supposed to wait until after the wedding and then they were going to look for a place to buy together," Adam said. "But two weeks ago she gets this brilliant idea, while we're all standing in line waiting to buy popcorn, that we should all start living together, like, *now,* and she invites Jerry and his daughters to move in with us, just like that, in the lobby of the multiplex. And when I start freaking out, she says, 'Oh, don't worry, everything's going to be great.' For her, maybe. Not for me."

"What's Jerry like?"

"Jerry's a nice guy, but his daughters are a pain; they take forever in the bathroom, they're all over the place, I can't walk around in, you know, the way I used to. Jerry's not the problem; my mom's the problem. Nothing seems to bother her; I mean, she's clueless. I don't know how to get through to her. She says she's all concerned that I've got this OCD thing, but she's, like, 'Oh, you'll go to the doctor and everything will be fine.' All she ever wants to hear is that I'm okay. I wish I could tell her what's really going on, but I can't. If she doesn't want to know about something, forget it—it's like talking to a wall."

The therapist asked Adam if he thought it might be helpful to have his mother join him for a session. Adam said it was okay with him but he doubted it would do any good.

A week later, Renée and Adam arrived at the office. Well dressed and carefully groomed, Renée looked as if she were in her early forties. She worked for a company that manufactured high-end cookware that she demonstrated and sold at gatherings in women's homes. She was energetic and friendly, and you could see how she would be successful at a career that required an outgoing, persuasive personality.

"So, how do we start?" she asked. Adam studied his lap. The therapist spoke.

"Adam, do you want to tell your mom what we've been talking about?"

"You mean about Jerry moving in and stuff?" Adam spoke without raising his eyes.

Renée looked puzzled. "I thought we were here to talk about Adam's problem," she said.

"Well, Mom, that *is* my problem," Adam said.

"Adam, you had a problem long before I even met Jerry. And we've been over this a million times. It just doesn't make sense for Jerry to renew his lease for another year when we're getting married in seven months." Renée looked at her son. "I explained this all to you, honey. We're going to need a bigger place in seven months anyway. The housing market is horrible, and if we try to sell the house now we'd lose at least fifty grand, maybe seventy-five. That's college tuition, right there."

"Yeah, Mom, but I'm not marrying the guy, you are. Your life is just the way you want it, and my life is ruined. Why can't I go live with Dad?"

"First of all, your life is not ruined. Second of all, you haven't exactly been easy to live with the last year. Do you really think your father is the best person for you to be with right now?" Adam was silent.

"It sounds as if the divorce has been hard on your son," the therapist said.

"Yes, it has, but it's been hard on me, too. And Jerry is a really good person. Let me tell you what kind of man this is. I had all these errands to run yesterday—it was getting late, and I desperately needed a jar of sundried tomatoes for a recipe I was doing—I had a show last night at a house on the other side of town—so I jumped in the car and, just my luck, I was really low on gas. But people are always saying there's some gas left even when the needle's on E, so I drove to the market and of course they were out of the kind in olive oil, which was the kind I needed. So I drove to another market five miles out of my way, and guess what? I ran out of gas. That's the kind of luck I have. I couldn't call the auto club, because you know how long that can take and the show was starting in less than an hour. So I called Jerry, and do you know, he was there in fifteen minutes. That's the kind of man he is." She looked at her son. "He's a good man, honey; you just have to give him a chance. I know this isn't easy for you, but it isn't easy for any of us. You're not the only one who has to adjust. You have to make an effort to pull yourself together."

Adam's head shot up. "Like I haven't been trying? Jeez, Mom, you don't just pull yourself together out of OCD. It's not like I can stop—I would if I could. It's, like, a disorder, okay? It's a real anxiety thing, not a bad mood or something I can just fix because you want me to. You don't know what it's like."

"No, I don't know what it's like. I'm sorry, but I can't relate to all this anxiety stuff. I'm just not an anxious person."

That wasn't how Adam's therapist saw it when she presented the case at one of our staff conferences.

According to the therapist, Renée appeared to be one of those people who was both profoundly self-involved yet minimally introspective, wrapped up in her own excitement and blind to the emotions, anxiety among them, roiling under her busy surface. Renée came off as gregarious and personable, but her inability to empathize with her son's distress revealed another side of her. Like many people with narcissistic tendencies, Renée was simultaneously aware of her feelings and unaware of the deeper forces driving those feelings.

Take her sundried tomato adventure. It wasn't bad luck that caused Renée to run out of gas but her anxiety about being late for a professional obligation. She knew her tank was nearly empty but she didn't want to be late, so when the anxiety kicked in, she acted impulsively and barreled on to not one market but two and then decried her bad luck when she ran out of gas.

Renée's invitation to Jerry and his daughters to move in was yet another reflexive-impulsive anxiety response. Feeling their wedding day growing closer and becoming increasingly panicky at the prospect of losing money on her house sale, she blurted out the invitation. Renée responded impulsively to relieve her own anxiety but, in so doing, greatly aggravated her son's.

The behavior wasn't new; as the therapist came to learn, Renée had been relating to anxiety in a reflexive-impulsive way for a long time. Adam described how, years earlier, his mother had blurted out at the dinner table that she couldn't take him to soccer practice the next day because she had to go in for a test to see if she had cancer and that the whole family was distraught for two weeks until the test came back negative. When the therapist asked Renée about this privately, a look of disbelief crossed Renée's face.

"I haven't thought about that for years!" she said. "It was no big deal. My gynecologist phoned to say that the results of my Pap test were inconclusive and that I should come back for another one to make sure everything was okay. It was nothing; everything was negative. But I'm amazed that Adam remembers that—he was only about eight or nine. I didn't even realize he understood what was going on." When the therapist described this episode, it seemed clear to me that Renée's impulsive announcement at the dinner table had been a reflexive response to her anxiety: it had relieved the anxiety she was feeling but burdened her loved ones with it.

Upon first reading about this case, it is difficult not to be judgmental about Renée's lack of empathy for Adam, as well as her lack of insight into how she was contributing to his distress. Was she really as callous and narcissistic as she came across, or was she reacting to Adam's therapy session the way she reacted whenever she felt uncomfortable or threatened by automatically and impulsively deflecting criticism and spinning the conversation to alleviate her anxiety and guilt?

I don't think that Renée was oblivious to her son's feelings; rather, I believe she was most likely running on automatic pilot, doing what she needed to in the moment to escape her anxious feelings. Her remark that she couldn't relate to Adam's anxiety because she didn't have any herself shows that she was at least as oblivious to her own issues as she was to her son's: how could she empathize with his anxiety when she was so detached from her own?

This isn't unusual in therapy: a family member sometimes comes in with the patient, and we realize that he or she needs treatment as much as the patient does—sometimes more. Had we been able to treat Renée, we would have worked to get her to understand that the anxiety she didn't think she had was adversely affecting the people around her, including herself. I believe that had Renée been aware of the role that anxiety played in her life, she would have embraced the chance to defuse it more thoughtfully. She might then have been able to see how her own anxiety was exacerbating Adam's OCD symptoms—which, you may recall, worsened after she impulsively invited Jerry and his daughters to move in—and modify her responses to aid in his recovery. Doing this would, I believe, have gone a long way toward helping Adam get a better handle on his OCD, as well as healing the dynamics of their relationship.

Renée and Teresa illustrate two different manifestations of a reflexive-impulsive anxiety relationship. Unlike Renée, Teresa was aware that she was having difficulty handling her anxiety and decided, after our serendipitous meeting on the plane, to face it head-on. After only a handful of therapy sessions she was able to identify the triggers that were creating the emotional chaos that affected her sleep and personal relationships. She wasn't afraid to search within herself and recognize that what she wasn't able to see for herself was as critical to her well-being as what she could see. Teresa continued to check in with me from time to time when she was in town, reporting on her progress, setbacks, and new goals. The last time I saw her was shortly after her father died, a time when it would have been understandable if some old behavior patterns had resurfaced. But she had become so aware of her tendency to react automatically that she had built in controls to be sure she got adequate sleep, exercise, and nutrition. Sure, she slipped up from time to time, but her actions were seldom unconscious. "It's those diaries that keep me steady," she said. "I'm still using them. Forcing myself to write down what I'm doing every day—okay, almost every day—is like having a light shining on me all the time so I can't backslide. It's a pain, but look: no more circles under my eyes!"

The questionnaire that follows is not a diagnostic tool but rather an exercise designed to help you determine if you may be relating to your anxiety in a reflexive-impulsive way. If you put some thought into answering the questions honestly, they may help you think about your anxiety in new ways.

MIGHT I HAVE A REFLEXIVE-IMPULSIVE RELATIONSHIP WITH MY ANXIETY?

1. When you find yourself in a stressful situation, do you tend to respond automatically, without thinking first?
2. Do you attempt to resolve most issues by taking action immediately, even before analyzing the consequences of your actions?
3. Are you more comfortable making decisions spontaneously than spending some time exploring options?
4. Are there actions you take or behaviors you manifest to relieve anxiety, even though such actions and behaviors may cause subsequent problems for you or others?
5. Do you wish you could have more control over your behavior when you are anxious?
6. How well does this relationship work for you?
   a. Positive aspects:

   b. Negative aspects:

five

THE PERVASIVE-ADAPTIVE RELATIONSHIP

Pervasive: diffused or spread through every part of

Adaptive: adjusting oneself to particular conditions or ways

At the heart of the pervasive-adaptive relationship is the sense that anxiety is an inherent part of the self, that you just wouldn't be you if you didn't have a slightly apprehensive, always-on-your-guard approach to life. People who relate to their anxiety in this way typically perceive their anxiousness as a personality trait, something they were born with. They say, "It's just the way I am" or "I've always been this way." In many cases they describe anxiety—or worrying or nervousness or intensity—as one of their defining qualities, if not the dominant one. Some even say that they would not be as successful as they are were it not for the nervous current beneath their skin. It is as if they have incorporated the anxiety into their résumé and view it, whether they know it or not, as a valuable component of their competence.

This is where the adaptive part comes in. In response to their pervasive anxious feelings, people involved in this relationship typically do things and make choices that accommodate their anxiety and may even capitalize on it. For example, a medical student with this relationship may feel most vital and at home in the emergency room and decide to spend her career there without realizing that her ability to think and perform well under pressure is a happy side effect of the buzz of anxiety that is always vibrating in her head. Just as some people have trouble concentrating when they are anxious, others, like this medical student, feel ultra-alert and focused. A narcotics agent who once came in for treatment and who had retired after years of international undercover work attributed her success in no small measure to the ingrained anxiety that had kept her alert and vigilant when her life depended on it, even though she did not realize it while she was working. I want to emphasize that in neither case was the woman's career choice a conscious accommodation to her anxious nature but rather a logical decision grounded in doing a certain kind of work in a certain kind of environment that felt like a good fit.

This is not to say that pervasive-adaptive relaters are by definition unaware of the connection between their anxiety and the way they live their lives; you can be skilled at deliberately making anxiety-accommodating decisions and still be part of this group. The defining characteristics of this category are that its members perceive their anxiety as an inextricable part of who they are and adapt to accommodate its presence in their lives, whether they know it or not.

All this may be well and good and often is, especially if the person making the accommodations channels her anxiety productively. Someone with a job that requires attention to detail—say, a file clerk or a researcher or an accountant—may make a practice of checking her work frequently and earn a reputation for reliability. But if she doesn't direct her anxiety effectively, it may breach the levees and flow into areas where it is not helpful. For example, someone in a supervisory position may expect subordinates to achieve her level of excellence, thus earning a reputation for being difficult to please and impossible to work for. Or she may be reluctant to delegate tasks to subordinates for fear they won't perform up to her standards, thus overburdening herself with work that others should be doing. At the other extreme is the supervisor who overdelegates to avoid anxiety, coaxing subordinates into taking assignments she is uncomfortable handling herself. For example, an executive who is nervous about speaking in public might urge a junior colleague to substitute for her at a talk she has promised to give, bestowing the assignment as if it were a gift—"I would like you to have this opportunity, Casey; it'll be a great experience for you"—when she is reaping the benefit of her ostensible largesse as much as her subordinate is. This is not necessarily a problem: in this case, the executive eludes an anxiety-provoking commitment and her subordinate gets an opportunity to hone his or her speaking skills. A problem arises when the executive is unable to adapt her circumstances to calm the anxiety and it escalates to a troublesome level, leaving her either known as the boss from hell, swamped with work, or habitually manipulating others to camouflage her vulnerabilities.

There are other ways this relationship can backfire on the job. I once knew a young woman who dealt with her anxiety by becoming a chronic pleaser. An entry-level employee in a market research firm, she was so worried about not being a star performer that she became a needy one, eager to show her supervisor how hard she was working and be reassured that her efforts were adequate. After she completed a task, she would hover around him and say things like "That analysis I did—was it okay?" or "Were you happy with the report I wrote?" He eventually grew reluctant to give her assignments and suggest improvements because he was afraid of causing her stress or hurting her feelings. They eventually parted ways, with both sides losing something in the process. "It's too bad," her boss said. "She had great skills, but it was exhausting to work with her." As for the young woman, her misdirected anxiety secured her the very rejection she was trying so hard to avoid.

If it is exhausting to work with a pervasive-adaptive relater, it can also be difficult to live with one—or not, depending on the interpersonal dynamics of the people involved. Some pervasive-adaptive relaters will find themselves eagerly pursued by, and earn the gratitude of, romantic partners who are only too happy to cede responsibility for running the household and tending the relationship. For example, a pervasive-adaptive relater's anxiety might manifest as an urge to confer order and discipline: she might structure the relationship by defining roles and responsibilities and would probably prefer a household organized just so and take charge of keeping it that way. Depending on who she's living with, this could be either a relief or a disaster. Her partner may cherish her as an antidote to his own disorganization, but if he (or she) wants to occasionally change a routine or household procedure, as most of us do, the pervasive-adaptive partner is likely to resist and find herself persona non grata. Such people are usually baffled by the irritation they inspire in others; in their minds, they are only trying to keep things organized and running smoothly. Although they are often sufficiently self-aware to know that they keep their anxiety at bay by controlling the way things are done, they are seldom aware that this is tantamount to controlling other people as well.

At the other extreme is the person who channels her anxiety into being a pleaser in her personal relationships, as the young market researcher did in her professional one. Agreeable and acquiescent, these people seldom express an opinion about where to go, what to do, or how to handle things and are seemingly content to go along with what everyone else decides. But unlike truly easygoing types, who don't give a hoot about participating in this sort of decision making, people who try to please others to quell their anxiety actually do have preferences but are too anxious to voice them. Rather than risk incurring the displeasure of others, they squelch their own desires and gain a reputation for being compliant. Mildly anxious, high-functioning people often have no shortage of companions who find them charming to be around, at least at the beginning. But the charm can wear thin as the anxiousness emerges from behind their affable veneers. They often require reassurance in even the most mundane interactions, as when, for example, you offer them a ride or the last piece of cake and they repeatedly ask, "Are you sure? Are you sure?" until you weary of the exchange and are tempted to withdraw the offer. And living with someone whose anxiety prompts her to always acquiesce and please can be just as burdensome as living with a control freak in that the more assertive partner always feels obligated to take charge and make the decisions.

Of course, you don't have to be sharing a household with a pervasive-adaptive relater to be affected by her anxiety. I know a person who is so averse to taking risks that she won't go out to dinner without researching the restaurants under consideration and checking out their menus, décor, prices, atmosphere—not a terrible thing, to be sure, but when you want to get together with someone like that, planning the event requires more phone calls and emails than seem necessary. Nor, of course, will you ever share with this person the pleasure of discovering a terrific new place. But for her, that's the point; she has adapted her anxiety toward averting the discomfort of an unpleasant surprise: the more she learns about something, the more likely she is to have a satisfactory outcome. Is this a bad trait? Not in this woman's case; she has managed to channel her anxiety in a way that works for her and the people around her, at least most of the time. She is renowned among her friends as an information junkie whose research benefits them in myriad ways, and her husband has no complaints, as they seldom have a bad meal when they dine out.

The bottom line is that if you have a pervasive-adaptive relationship with your anxiety, it will work best if you are conscious of when you are acting in response to your anxiety and can channel it in a direction that is potentially beneficial to you and perhaps even to others. If the anxiety has nowhere productive to go, it is bound to surface in a different—and probably unexpected—way.

LESLIE: "I DIDN'T THINK I COULD BE ANY OTHER WAY"

"This is crazy—it just isn't me to worry this way. I stare at myself in the mirror sometimes because I feel so different inside, I figure I must have changed on the outside, too."

Leslie was adamant: something fundamental about her had changed. She used to be fearless, priding herself on her lack of concern about things other people worried about. In her twelve-year career as an investigative reporter at a large U.S. newspaper, she became known for her tough interviewing style and willingness to go after big shots when pursuing a lead. She thrived on the adrenaline rush of digging up the shady deal, the secret payoff, the telltale email that exposed wrongdoing and got the bad guys in trouble. By the time she met Trevor, a lawyer whom she eventually married, she was thirty-four, had traveled all over the country, and made no secret of the fact that her apartment had no furniture in it except a television and a futon: there was no point in furnishing the place, she told him, because she was hardly ever there.

But now Leslie was awash in anxiety. At thirty-nine, she had been married to Trevor for nearly five years and was the mother of a four-year-old girl she doted upon. She had not worked as a journalist since Peyton was born; after taking three months' maternity leave, she had felt uneasy at the thought of leaving the child in someone else's care and gone on an extended leave of absence. She said she enjoyed being a full-time mother more than she'd thought she would; whereas some stay-at-home moms she knew spoke of feeling overwhelmed with all they had to do, Leslie was undaunted. She joined the preschool's board of directors and volunteered to serve as chair of its annual fund-raising auction, agreed to edit the neighborhood newsletter, and hosted a play group at her house one morning a week. When people heard about her journalism career and asked her if she missed it, she said she certainly didn't miss the relentless pressure of newspaper work. She said she enjoyed the tranquillity of her life: she didn't have to worry about paying the mortgage on time or at all; in fact, she was living in more luxurious circumstances than she had ever imagined she would. Leslie said, somewhat self-consciously, that her husband came from an "established"—code for "wealthy"—New England family and that, although the house she lived in with him and Peyton sometimes felt too grand, after so many years of living like a nomad, it felt good to have a real home.

That's why Leslie was baffled by her anxiousness. She'd never had anxiety problems when she was zipping around the country, meeting deadlines, pleasing editors, and coming home to a microwaved frozen entrée for dinner. Why should she be anxious now, when her life was so much more secure?

"Ten years ago, it would have made sense for me to be sitting here," she said. "I was flying all over the place, running all the time, couldn't commit to anyone. I thrived on relationships that meant nothing and ended before they really began, which was fine with me; I didn't want to choose between my work and a boyfriend. I do remember sometimes having a fantasy of coming home to a loving man and someone calling me 'Mommy'—not the same person, of course—and thinking someday maybe I'd also have a normal life. Now I have exactly that: a husband who provides for me better than I could ever have dreamed and a wonderful daughter, whom I love more than anything.

"So why do I feel edgy so much of the time? For the past six months I've had this nonstop anxiety, only there's really nothing to be anxious about. When I was working and under all that pressure, I don't remember feeling nearly as freaked out as I do now. I've also started having stomach problems for the first time in years. I was diagnosed with irritable bowel syndrome when I was a freshman in college, but they said it was probably stress-related, and I didn't have it when I was working, so why would I have it now? You know, I've never missed a deadline—I even went into labor on my due date—and yet now, when I'm calling all the shots, I sometimes start worrying as if I'm paranoid.

"My daughter just turned four and is absolutely fine. Not a thing wrong with her. But whenever Peyton doesn't feel well, I feel I have to take her to the doctor just to make sure there's nothing seriously wrong. Even if I know that half the preschool is down with a bug, I still feel that maybe she's got something different from the other kids or it will affect her differently than it did the other kids. And when we're at the doctor's I'm still worrying: What if he misses something? What if he prescribes something and she has an allergic reaction? I ask lots of questions and write everything down so I can research it when I get home. I'm a reporter, right? That's what I do. Except the last time we were there the pediatrician said something like 'I'd better watch what I say or I'll end up on the front page,' and I realized I was making him uncomfortable. Then he gave Peyton a prescription for antibiotics, so when we got home I went on the Web to check out side effects and ended up staying online until two in the morning reading about the hazards of antibiotic immunity. I kept thinking, This isn't going to happen to Peyton; she doesn't take antibiotics often enough to become immune to them. But you read all these horror stories about kids getting sick with a harmless bug but the medications don't work, and before you know it, they're on life support.

"I just can't stop worrying about her. And now I'm worrying about me. Take food: I never had a weight problem because I often forgot to eat when I was doing a story. Sometimes I wouldn't realize until six or seven at night that I hadn't eaten, and then only because I would hear my stomach growling on my interview tapes. I'd get to my hotel in the middle of the night and everything would be closed and I'd scrounge around in my bag for half a granola bar or bum an apple from the front desk and that would be dinner. But now I'm obsessed with food. I rummage through the pantry checking expiration dates, and I worry if there's an E. coli outbreak or a beef recall. I try to eat regular meals, but sometimes I feel so bloated that I can't stand the thought of putting anything in my stomach. And when I do start to get hungry, I sometimes get anxious, like when I was pregnant, and I start thinking, What if there isn't any food available? What if I don't eat and I pass out while I'm driving with Peyton in the car? It sounds ridiculous as I say it, but when it's happening it feels totally real. And what's real about it is not the certainty that calamity will strike, because I know that it probably won't, but what feels real is that it's my job, my responsibility, my mission to keep calamity from striking. Because if something happens to me, who will take care of Peyton? Sure, she'd have Trevor, but he works all the time, and I can't see him changing that even if I weren't there. I'm her mother, after all."

When I asked Leslie if she had any recollection of being anxious as a child, she said no but, when pressed, admitted that she had bitten her nails until she was a senior in high school. And there were also her irritable bowel symptoms, which she said had gone away for the most part after she graduated and started working.

"You know," she said, "now that I think about it, maybe it is the IBS kicking in again. But why should it hit now after all these years? That's really weird."

Actually, it wasn't weird. Irritable bowel syndrome, also known as spastic colon, is a gastrointestinal disorder that affects 10 to 20 percent of the population and nearly twice as many women as men. Symptoms typically include constipation, diarrhea, bloating, and abdominal pain and seem to be triggered in many people by anxiety, stress, and feelings of guilt and resentment.[1] In a study at the Medical University of South Carolina, researchers found that while fewer than half of people suffering from IBS sought treatment, between 50 and 90 percent of those who did seek treatment were also suffering from one or more anxiety problems, including social anxiety disorder, panic disorder, PTSD, and GAD.[2] In another study at the State University of New York Health Science Center, researchers found that more than 46 percent of the participants who had panic disorder also had IBS.[3]

Given Leslie's history of IBS and her exaggerated worry about Peyton's well-being (as well as her own), it wasn't surprising to hear she was having stomach problems. What was surprising was the intense physical response she was having to ordinary mother angst. Anyone hearing about this case would know that Leslie's worries about her daughter were normal for a new parent; both mothers and fathers of young children are often appalled by the threats they suddenly perceive lurking everywhere: bathtubs, kitchen knives, staircases, under-sink cabinets, and cars present opportunities for horrors they never thought of before. Moreover, new parents are commonly beset by intimations of their own mortality and grapple with thoughts of what might happen to their child if they should suddenly be gone for good. But these worries typically abate with time, and in Leslie's case, they didn't.

Then one day it came to me: Leslie's anxiety may have been focused on her child, but it was not there *because* of her child. Rather, Leslie's anxiety was a long-standing and pervasive element of her personality, to which she had skillfully adapted by choosing a profession that enabled her to channel it productively. We know that Leslie was anxious as a child and young adult, so it is plausible to infer that her anxiety predated the birth of her child. It is also safe to infer that she had not chosen her career based on a careful analysis of her temperament. Rather, she had chosen reporting because the urgency of journalism appealed to her yen for excitement and felt like a good fit.

Leslie had adapted superbly to her anxiety—that is, until she went on hiatus from her career. This woman went from talking to dozens of people a day and doing intellectually demanding work on a tight schedule to focusing her energies on caring for a young, dependent child and having limited opportunities for adult interaction. The hectic quality of journalism offered her virtually unlimited venues for channeling her anxiety; the repetitive, predictable practice of motherhood provided very few. Leslie channeled some anxious energy into her volunteer activities—her worries and IBS symptoms had abated somewhat while she was running the fund-raiser, which was a big, big job—but once that outlet disappeared, her anxiety had nowhere to go but into overdrive.

Leslie is a nearly perfect example of someone with a pervasive-adaptive anxiety relationship: her anxious feelings were so much a part of her that she experienced them as an essential component of her being. It never occurred to her that her intensity was fueled by anxiety, nor that it was anxiety that enabled her to sometimes go all day without eating or all night without sleeping. Leslie did not experience her anxiety as such, but rather as having an energy level that was as relentlessly high as her appetite was low; it was just the way she was. Which is not to say she didn't feel the anxiety—she did—but she didn't think she was anxious; to her, her edgy exuberance was as much a part of her Leslie-ness as her straight hair and staccato laugh.

"I didn't think there was any other way to be," she said. "People used to ask me where I got all my energy and how I could work so late into the night, and I kept thinking, How can you *not* have all this energy? How can you fall asleep at ten o'clock?, because I'd never been able to turn off the vibration. It was always there, it was just the way I was. It never occurred to me that I could be any other way."

Which brings me to my next point: I am not suggesting that Leslie *should* be any other way. There's a lot to be said for approaching life with energy and enthusiasm and a buzz as long as you recognize the source of the commotion. What I am suggesting—all right, advocating—is that you develop an awareness of the buzz and the shimmy that are rattling your cage and consider the possibility that low-level anxiety may be a pervasive element of your consciousness. Once you do that, you can identify the ways you have adapted to the anxiety and evaluate whether or not they are working for you.

In Leslie's case, her outside-the-home career adaptations were superb, but when she stopped working, her abundant energy and intensity had nowhere to go. When she started therapy, Leslie began to recognize that her old adaptations—always running, rushing to meet deadlines, living on the edge—were inconsistent with her new life. At first she thought she had to come up with activities that would keep her busy, but she soon found that editing a quarterly newsletter and hosting a weekly play group weren't going to do it: the demands these activities exerted were insufficient to accommodate her anxiety output. Leslie needed not to raise her activity level but to raise her awareness that her anxiety had always been there; it was her successful adaptation to it that had kept it at bay. Now, with that former adaptation no longer operational, she had to readapt and find new ways to creatively channel her anxiety.

My goal for Leslie was for her not to do more but rather to *be* more: I wanted her to do things that would enable her to just be present with her anxiety, befriend it, and adapt anew in ways that would channel it successfully. She decided to stop by a martial arts studio near her home—it offered tai chi as well as tae kwon do—and sign up for an introductory class to see how she liked it. She also agreed to drop by a local yoga studio and look into trying an ashtanga yoga class, which is both physically and mentally challenging. I persuaded her to let me lend her a guided meditation CD, which took some doing—Leslie didn't think she'd have the patience to sit still long enough to use it—but I got her to commit to doing at least fifteen minutes' worth at least three times before her next session. I neither expected nor wanted her to commit to all these activities; my goal was, of course, to motivate her to think in new ways about her anxiety and try new ways of adapting to it. When I saw her last, she had nixed the meditation but was doing ashtanga yoga three times a week. "It's killing me," she said, "but I love it. I'm so strung out after class, I don't have the energy to worry."

JORDANA: "ANXIETY MAKES ME GOOD AT WHAT I DO—WITHOUT IT, I'D BE LIKE EVERYBODY ELSE"

I first met Jordana at an early-morning aerobics class I went to when I was single. The class, made up of professionals working out before work, was mostly female and entirely sleep-deprived. Afterward, we'd shower, gather at the mirror, and share news about our jobs, families, and love lives.

We were always hurrying and doing several things at once, but none of us could multitask like Jordana. She would fly around the locker room, yanking up her pantyhose and working gel through her dark spiky hair while delivering hilarious anecdotes about life as a music teacher and choral director in an inner-city middle school. She was always in a rush and frequently dashed into class late, dropping her stuff and taking a spot at the back of the room. When she learned what I did for a living, she whooped with delight. "You could have a field day with me," she said. "When it comes to anxiety, I'm right up there with the greats."

Jordana was in her late forties but looked at least a decade younger. Petite, energetic, and very attractive, she charmed us with her self-deprecating sense of humor and kept us hysterical with stories from school, such as the time they had been on a bus en route to an out-of-state choral competition and three sopranos had thrown up on the altos; the time a baritone had toppled off a riser in the middle of "Ol' Man River"; and my favorite, the time she had sent fifty kids home with permission slips for a field trip to New York City's Times Square to see *The **Loin** King*.

"It's always something," she'd say. "I'm always running late and I end up rushing around and screwing up. The other morning Chico spat up a hair ball on the white carpet and it took me fifteen minutes to clean it up and then I couldn't find my earring and spent ten minutes looking for that. So what are my choices? Do I leave the cat mess and worry all day about the carpet getting stained, or do I take the time to clean it and have a heart attack because I'm late for work? Do I spend the day worrying that I've lost a diamond earring, or do I take the time to look for it and make myself late again?" Jordana said she couldn't leave the house until everything was just so, so it was hard to get out on time—missing eyeglasses or car keys, mopping the kitchen floor, scrubbing the shower stall, closing the curtains throughout the apartment, phone calls from students—all these things conspired to make her late. When I asked how students got her home number, Jordana said she gave it to them because she felt it was her responsibility to be reachable. "These kids don't have a lot going on, and the chorus means a lot to them," she said. "They need to know they can count on me to be there for them twenty-four–seven."

Jordana, who had never been married, had been involved with her current beau for several years. Glenn was a composer and arranger who had been living apart from his wife for five years but had not yet secured a divorce, ostensibly because his wife's part-time job didn't provide her with health benefits and she needed to remain on his insurance policy as long as possible. It was easy to see this as the same old story: man with no intention of divorcing his wife misleads gullible single woman into thinking he will soon be free. But it was more complicated than that. One moment Jordana would sound bitter at still being single, but the next she'd say she really wasn't in a rush for Glenn's divorce to come through.

"I can be neurotic and work all the time, especially if we're preparing for a concert," she said. "I couldn't do that if I were living with someone. This way, if I feel I need to work, I can call Glenn and cancel at the last minute."

"Why do you feel it's okay to cancel at the last minute when you've got a commitment to see each other?" I asked.

"It's not as if he's committed to me, is it? Anyway, it's better this way. Glenn's an emotional guy; he always wants to talk about the relationship and how he's feeling and where it's going. And sometimes I just want to be by myself and get my work done. There's always something I can be doing for school, and he doesn't understand how anxious I get if I don't feel prepared. He doesn't get that I can't sleep at night unless everything is done. Talk about anxiety! Every kid has a folder with their name on it with the music arranged in the order that we sing the pieces. Every night before I go home I check all the folders and make sure everyone has the right music and that nothing has gotten lost. I don't get home until late, and then I've got to feed Chico and maybe myself, and then I'm on the Internet until one or two in the morning printing stuff—I like to put something new in their folders every day. A few weeks ago I was up until three. It's like I can't stop; I've got to keep going until I've done everything I can to make things perfect.

"The kids need me. No one has done with those kids what I've been able to do—no one. They don't have much that they feel good about except for singing, and it takes a lot to keep that going. Sure, I've got a lot of anxiety. But if I weren't so anxious, I'd be just like everyone else: I'd have them do a few songs, and that would be the end of it."

"You sound like an amazing teacher," I said, "but it also sounds as if you're working around the clock. When do you have time to do anything else?"

"I don't," she said. "I see Glenn sometimes but hardly anyone else. I used to go out with friends, but I don't hear from a lot of them anymore. I talk all day at work, and I simply cannot face talking on the phone at night. So when people leave me messages, I don't call them back a lot of the time. And a lot of them don't call me anymore."

"And are you okay with that?"

Jordana didn't answer for a while. "No, I guess not, but what can I do? I'm on my own—I don't have a husband paying the mortgage and the bills. I need to put money away for when I retire. I have to work hard because it's just me."

This was a long time ago, and I'm sure there are some things I'm forgetting. But looking back, I see now that Jordana had a pervasive-adaptive relationship with her anxiety. Unlike Leslie, Jordana was aware that a current of anxiety vibrated beneath the surface of her life and consciously regarded it as an essential element of her identity and professional success. This is all to the good: each of us lives with a certain amount of anxiety, and it can be beneficial if we make it work for us.

But the pervasiveness of Jordana's anxiety also caused her to adapt in some ways that, I believe, mitigated her happiness. It caused her to withdraw from her friends and family, depriving her of both companionship and safe environments in which to blow off steam. And, unlike Leslie, who was able to forge an intimacy with a man, commit to him, and start a family, Jordana's anxiety impeded her romance from growing into something more. Though Glenn may have been legally unavailable to marry Jordana, she in turn seemed emotionally unavailable to him. I imagine that, had Glenn shown up one night with a bottle of Champagne in one hand and a divorce decree in the other, Jordana's anxiety would likely have outspiraled her joy.

Let me make something clear: I'm not saying that Jordana's happiness would have been sealed had she married Glenn, nor am I suggesting that marriage is a panacea for whatever ails you. What I am saying is that I believe Jordana would have been happier had her anxiety not fueled her relentless work regimen and interfered with her ability to connect with friends, family, and lover alike. As I see it, her life lacked balance—that elusive quality—and she was suffering for it. And though some workaholics might argue that balance is an overrated virtue, I would argue back that, for most people, it's hard to overrate the virtues, both physical and psychological, of connecting with others.

The nature of a pervasive-adaptive anxiety relationship implies a lack of boundaries, which is how the anxiety becomes pervasive in the first place. In this relationship, the anxiety is not a response to a stimulus and so does not subside when the stimulus is removed. Instead, it vibrates nonstop in the body and mind and seeps into every corner of our consciousness, redrawing our map of the world and distorting the boundaries that preserve the inner self from its outward identities and obligations. If you relate to your anxiety in this way, you probably have difficulty, as Jordana did, setting boundaries that protect you from feeling pulled in numerous directions at once. I'm not talking about the occasional conflict that makes you weigh alternatives and choose between them, such as how you might feel upon receiving two appealing dinner invitations for the same night. Rather, I refer to a nagging feeling that, no matter which invitation you accept, persuades you that you really should have chosen the other or even neither, in favor of doing something else that you feel you *ought* to do.

Looking back with hindsight's perfect vision, I see that working all the time and making herself so available to her students was Jordana's way of adapting to her pervasive anxiety; so was maintaining an exaggerated orderliness that required her to ensure her house was just so and everything was present and accounted for—including misplaced jewelry—before she left in the morning. She was always busy working and perfecting her environment because focusing on those goals, which can never be completely achieved, distracted her from the anxiousness that was always vibrating within her. I also see now that Jordana's romantic woes were partly of her own making. At the time, I commiserated with what I believed was her dismay at being involved with a man who wouldn't commit to her, but now I see she was complicit in paralyzing the romance's momentum. Jordana's withdrawal from Glenn, her family, and her friends balanced in an undesirable way her ultra-availability at work: in giving everything to her students, she had little left for her other, more intimate relationships.

Yes, dealing with a difficult supervisor or colleague can take it out of you—no question. But in the grand scheme of things, it takes more effort to conduct ongoing relationships with parents, siblings, a spouse, children, and friends than with colleagues because personal obligations usually ask more of us than do professional ones. The boundaries that define personal relationships are more fluid than those at work and require more frequent examination and renewal. This takes time and energy, two commodities that Jordana had in short supply. I believe, in the end, that Jordana was too exhausted to engage fully in personal intimacies and so let them wither.

Many of us can see pieces of our own personalities here. Who hasn't cleaned out a closet after a tough day at the office and felt calmed by both the activity and the sense of order she created? How often have you agreed to go to a certain restaurant or movie even though you would have preferred another, simply because it was easier (and felt socially correct) to please the person inviting you than to suggest a different one? The key to making the pervasive-adaptive relationship (or any of the other ones) work for you is to be conscious of why you're doing what you're doing and be able to step aside and ask, "Is this working for me and the people I care about?" If the answer is yes, continue on your way. But if the answer is no, why not explore some different ways of reacting or responding to that inner buzz?

MIGHT I HAVE A PERVASIVE-ADAPTIVE RELATIONSHIP WITH MY ANXIETY?

1. Do you feel a constant, underlying anxiety, as if you are always on alert?
2. If so, do you believe that the anxiousness is an element of who you are, a part of your personality, as opposed to a reaction to events in your life?
3. If family members or friends were to describe you, would they use terms such as intense, high-strung, and/or high maintenance?
4. Do you find yourself doing things regularly to keep your anxiety at bay?

5. Does your need to always be in control affect your personal relationships, professional relationships, or both?
6. Does this anxiety relationship work for you?
   a. Positive aspects:

   b. Negative aspects:

six

THE PRIMITIVE-PREVENTIVE RELATIONSHIP

Primitive: of behavior, thought, or emotion originating in unconscious needs or desires and unaffected by objective reasoning

Preventive: designed to keep something undesirable such as illness, harm, or accidents from occurring

You know you have a primitive-preventive relationship when you adhere to regimens of anxiety-preventing behaviors in the hope that your vigilance will keep your anxiety under control. The anxious feelings themselves may be likened to a volatile husband: as long as you iron his shirts, keep the house clean, and have dinner on the table at the appointed time, he won't explode. Women with this kind of anxiety tend to devise schemes and rituals that enable them to manage their anxiety without confronting it.

If I had to choose two words to describe the primitive-preventive relationship, they would be "if" and "then": If I do this thing in just this way, then that thing that makes me anxious won't happen. As in:

"If I show up early for work every morning and turn my reports in before they're due, then I'll never have to worry about losing my job or running out of money."

"If I go to a college close to home, then I won't feel like I'm abandoning my parents."

"If I don't allow my child to eat sugary cereals or candy or drink soda, and if I make sure he eats only organic food, then maybe he won't get diabetes like me."

Each of these statements expresses a wish to forestall anxiety and proposes a way to do it. The fears—losing your livelihood and maybe your home, hurting your parents and perhaps losing their affection, harming your child's health—represent basic, primitive needs we all have: the need to provide food and shelter to ourselves and our families, the need to be loved, the need to nurture and protect our children. When we are anxious about these things, the anxiety feels deep and urgent, as if our very existence were on the line. Which is not to say our existence actually *is* on the line; the anxiety just *feels* that way. The feelings are not based on a rational appraisal of risk, nor can they be allayed by thinking things through. The feelings are elemental and instinctive, dark and irresistible, and they connect to our most basic human needs. That's the primitive part.

And the preventive part? As its name would suggest, the preventive part is the things we do to prevent these anxieties from snaking up our spines and shaking our foundations. I'm not speaking now of the things we do to prevent actual calamities from happening—for instance, fastening our seat belts to avoid hurtling through the windshield or locking the kitchen cabinets to prevent a toddler from getting into the Drāno. I'm speaking now of the things we do and choices we make to prevent or ease anxieties that are not literally life-threatening but feel like primal attacks to our physical or emotional well-being, because this part of the relationship is not about preventing actual harm but rather about soothing our feelings. A young woman who chooses her hairstyle, wardrobe, career, and fiancé to please her critical mother makes these choices in an attempt to prevent herself from feeling the primitive anxiety aroused by her mother's disapproval. A wife and mother who goes back to school to finish her doctorate but drops out because her husband and kids feel neglected subjugates her will to theirs to prevent feeling anxious about her household falling into disarray and being perceived as an incompetent homemaker and selfish wife and mother.

Neither the young woman trying to please her mother nor the mother trying to please her family would describe her anxiety as feeling life-threatening, but I imagine they both might feel as if they were, in some sense, fighting for their lives—their emotional lives, to be precise. Each of these women might admit that she was being inauthentic by shaping her life to conform to others' expectations, but I believe they would also claim they were doing so in the name of a higher cause, that cause being filial loyalty in the first case, womanly duty in the second. "My mother wants the best for me, so why shouldn't I try to please her?" the daughter might say; "I'd love to finish my degree, but it's really hard on my family and my family comes first," the wife and mother might say. The sacrifice and self-abnegation inherent in these statements are noble and understandable in light of the various obligations weighing on these women. But I would also argue that they are choosing sacrifice and self-abnegation to forestall the soul-wrenching anxiety they would experience were they to place their own fulfillment above that of their loved ones. The prospect of alienating a mother's affection and the idea of denying a husband and children the constant nurturing presence they have come to expect could easily, in my view, shake the foundations of a woman's sense of self and inspire feelings of chaos and terror. Why would she not choose to deny her own needs, however much disappointment she might feel, if doing so made her feel more secure in the affections of the people she held most dear? This is the essence of the primitive-preventive anxiety relationship: making choices and taking steps to prevent yourself from feeling anxiety that is too fundamental and too deep to talk yourself out of.

For most of us, the primitive instinct to preserve our loved ones and ourselves takes the form of everyday anxieties, which, intense though they may be at times, are traceable back to real and rational fears: "Look both ways before you cross the street! Don't play with matches! Don't talk to strangers!" But for some of us, primitive instincts manifest in irrational, abnormal fears known as phobias.

Take my friend Merle. It was at least twenty-five years ago that I found myself in New York, my hometown, on business. I had had a morning meeting on the West Side and called Merle from a pay phone (remember those?) to see if she could meet me for lunch. She suggested a café near her office on Madison Avenue and agreed to meet me in an hour. It was a balmy day, and I had just enough time for a leisurely stroll through Central Park, which seemed like a great idea, high heels and all. Along with the usual jugglers, mimes, musicians, and baby carriages was a cluster of people watching something. I squeezed into the crowd and saw a young man with a large snake coiled around his heavily tattooed arm and neck. I don't know what kind of snake it was, but I do remember its tongue darting out of its mouth and the crowd being absolutely mesmerized. I would have been, too, if I'd had more time, but I needed to get over to the East Side, so I paused only briefly.

When Merle showed up at the restaurant, I could barely contain myself. "Only in New York!" I said. "My first day back, and what should I see in Central Park but a young guy covered with tattoos and a snake wrapped around his body. I wish you could have seen it—"

"Eeeeuw! I don't!" Merle said. She grimaced, snapped open the menu, and busied herself with the specials of the day. End of conversation.

Five months later I was back in New York and called Merle again to make a lunch date.

"It's so warm for October, and I don't have much time. How about we get some sandwiches to go and eat them in the park?"

"Jerilyn," she said, "I haven't been in Central Park since you were here last time."

"What are you talking about? Don't you jog in the park?"

"Not since you told me about the snake, I don't." I knew Merle didn't like snakes—very few people do—but this sounded a bit extreme. Did Merle have a phobia?

We met up, bought some sandwiches, and settled onto a stone bench on Fifth Avenue just outside the wall bordering the park. I turned to my friend.

"Merle, I remember telling you about the snake guy, but I don't recall you saying anything about it. Why didn't you say something?"

"I didn't say anything because I wanted to block it out of my mind. But the next day I went to run in the park and I was convinced I'd see that guy and I couldn't go in. I know it's irrational: it's not like the snake was in the wild, and you said the guy was holding on to it. And Central Park is huge; I probably couldn't have found the guy if I'd tried. But none of that matters. Just knowing it was there is enough. I simply can't go into the park anymore."

It all began to make sense: the weekends we were supposed to go hiking and Merle ended up canceling, and the story she had told about having to leave in the middle of *Raiders of the Lost Ark* because of the snake pit scene. I suppose I had always known that Merle had an aversion to snakes. But I had never realized it was a specific phobia—an irrational fear and avoidance of a specific place, situation, or object (as distinguished from social phobia, a fear of being judged by others, or agoraphobia, a fear of public places or open spaces)—until the Central Park episode.

Some months later Merle and I ran into a mutual acquaintance who imported luxury leather goods and offered us a great deal if we would come up to his showroom and find something we liked. What woman would turn down a chance to get a great deal on a luxury bag? Neither of us, that's for sure, so we agreed to meet in the lobby of his building a few days later. As I walked in Merle saw me, waved me over to an elevator bank with "31–49" emblazoned on an illuminated display (this was back when you could still walk into a Manhattan office building without signing in), and pressed the button.

"He's on forty-two," she said.

Uh-oh.

I had come a long way with my height phobia and the days when I couldn't go higher than the tenth floor of a building. But the forty-second floor was pushing it.

"Yikes," I said. "Forty-two? I'm not sure I can do this." Merle knew about my height phobia, but that didn't stop her from looking at me as if I were insane.

"Jerilyn, that's ridiculous. We're inside. It's not as if we're going out onto a balcony."

"The balcony is irrelevant. The very idea of stepping out of an elevator onto the forty-second floor is the only thing that's relevant to me. It's totally irrational, and I know it's hard to understand—wait: Merle, think snakes. This is my snake."

"Oh, I get it," she said.

We did make it up to the showroom, and we did get our bargains. But the best deal for me that day was when I mustered the courage to look out the window, forty-two stories over Manhattan.

That was a long time ago, and Merle steadfastly maintains that her snake phobia hardly affects her life anymore. But when I spoke with her recently, her comments suggested otherwise. Outside of a foray to Shakespeare in the Park and an occasional visit to a restaurant within the park, Merle was still hobbled by her fear. In her words:

"I still dread going into the park. As crazy as it sounds, I'm still afraid I'll see a snake and have those feelings. And I won't see the *Raiders of the Lost Ark* sequel, either. We were supposed to go to Costa Rica last year, and I canceled the trip. I called the hotel, and the woman at the front desk assured me there were no snakes. But how could she really assure me? There's jungle everywhere down there. It's not that I'm afraid of getting a snakebite; I'm afraid of the snake. It's been the same since my childhood. When I was a girl, we had a huge dictionary with a colorful fold-out page of snakes. My sister used to chase me with that page, and I'd run around screaming. So it's been this way for a long time."

Even though Merle has a phobia and not everyday anxiety, I have included her here because she is a good example of someone with a primitive-preventive anxiety relationship. Her decisions to forgo hiking, abandon running in Central Park, and cancel a vacation to Costa Rica were preventive measures to protect her from her phobia of snakes, or ophidiophobia, one of the oldest and commonest aversions on the planet.

Of course, whereas anxiety about snakes and heights is connected to our most primitive fears, not all phobias are primitive in nature. I once had a patient who suffered from a phobia about anything to do with the state of Florida. It had gotten so bad that she had trouble shopping for groceries because of all the citrus fruit, orange juice, and cardboard palm trees on display. You're probably waiting for the punch line, but I'm not joking: this was a genuine phobia and not very funny for the patient, although, like many people with phobias, she could appreciate its absurdity. Still, as much as she was tormented by her phobia, I would not call it primitive: the anxiety she might experience due to, say, a televised glimpse of the Miami Dolphins or an episode of *Miami Vice,* however intense, did not issue from the primeval forest of her psyche, as did (and does) Merle's fear of snakes. It is the ancient, primordial nature of Merle's anxiety and the measures she takes to prevent it that places it in the primitive-preventive category. And, as we shall see, she is not alone.

CLAUDIA AND BERNICE: FEARFUL OF THEIR CHILDREN'S PAIN

If the urge to protect one's offspring is one of the most primitive known to man, it probably is *the* most primitive known to woman. It certainly was for Claudia and Bernice, who do not know each other but had something in common: an intense need to protect their children from pain. I'm not talking about the catastrophe-inspired adrenaline rush that enables a five-foot two-inch, 120-pound woman to pry a two-ton Buick off her child. What I'm talking about is a feeling of colossal anxiety that accompanies any intimation that your child may be suffering physical or psychological pain or discomfort, however minor. Though many of us would not hesitate to fling ourselves into harm's way to prevent a beloved child from incurring bodily harm (or marrying that ne'er-do-well she's been seeing), most of us would not go to extreme lengths to protect that child from, for example, the agony of having to wake up early enough to get to school on time.

But Claudia would. Claudia *did.*

When six-year-old Samantha came home with a note from her teacher complaining that she was chronically late for class, Claudia might have done any number of things. She might have made sure Samantha got out of bed at the appointed hour, put her to bed earlier, or threatened to send her to school in her pajamas if she didn't wake up early enough to get dressed. But Claudia did none of these things. Instead, she made an appointment with the teacher and let her know she wasn't about to stress out her child by making her get up before she was ready.

"I can't believe the nerve of that woman," Claudia told me at the time. "We pay a lot of money to send Samantha to that school, and they should be able to accommodate her. It's first grade, for heaven's sake; she's not going to miss anything that important, and she's way above grade level anyway. I don't want my kid to have to get up in the morning if she's tired."

As I write this, I cringe at how terrible it sounds. Claudia is in fact a good person and a lot of fun. She's very smart, has a great sense of humor, does a lot of community work, and is loyal to her many friends. But she's also paralyzed with anxiety whenever she anticipates that her children—she has three, all grown now—may be forced to endure hardship, pain, inconvenience, or discomfort. Every loving parent (and grandparent, stepparent, aunt, uncle, or guardian) wants to protect his or her kids from disappointment and unhappiness but can usually tolerate the kids' growing pains. Sometimes, when we're at our best, we can even embrace such trials as opportunities for children to develop strength, self-reliance, and moxie.

But Claudia couldn't do this. Whenever her babies cried, she picked them up immediately, and whenever they fussed, she acceded to their every whim. There were no bedtimes for the children, and they weren't required to eat what Claudia had cooked for dinner: if they didn't like mackerel, she'd make macaroni and cheese. Nor were they even required to eat; if they weren't hungry, they could pass on dinner and get takeout later. Leaving the kids with a sitter was out of the question. "I was afraid a babysitter wouldn't take proper care of the kids, so we never left them with anyone," she said. (To Claudia, of course, taking proper care of the kids meant allowing them to do whatever they wanted, whenever they wanted, however they wanted, which no sane sitter would agree to.) The mere idea that any of her children might feel hungry, lonely, disappointed, or sad evoked in Claudia a swell of anxiety so potent that to protect herself from the feelings, she determined never to impose on her children any rules, demands, or expectations that might make them unhappy. She says the roots of the anxiety took hold in her childhood. In her words:

"When I was growing up, my parents were busy and I had to take care of most of my needs. I wasn't mistreated but I've always felt emotionally neglected, so I decided that if I were ever a parent, I would make sure that I provided for all of my kids' emotional needs. When they were growing up, instead of allowing them to solve some of their own problems, I did it for them. Like crying themselves to sleep: when I heard even a whimper, I immediately came to their aid and comforted them rather than let them work it through. And with school—whenever they had an issue with a teacher about a late assignment or a bad grade, I came running to the rescue instead of making them talk to the teacher themselves. Gregory once came home all upset because the teacher assigned him to write a report about the Empire State Building, and we had just visited the Statue of Liberty and he really wanted to write about that. He was carrying on and begged me to talk to the teacher about it, so I called the teacher and got him to change the assignment. But what I should have done was tell Greg to talk to the teacher himself. That would have given him some experience dealing with authority figures, which would come in handy now. He's been working the same job now for three years without a raise. He complains about it all the time, but when I tell him he should go to his boss and demand a raise, he always has an excuse for why it won't do any good. And Connor, my baby—well, he might never have that problem because at the rate he's going, he'll be in college for the rest of his life. This business of me always coming to my children's aid didn't give them the tools to be able to cope with difficult situations. Looking back, I think it's really important to do that for your kids."

I should point out that Claudia was not feeling anxious because she believed her children to be in any real psychological or physical danger: if you had asked her at the time what permanent injury they might sustain were she, for example, to make them go without dinner one night, she would have reasonably told you that they would be hungry for a few hours and that would be all. What was not reasonable were the anxious feelings that would claw her at the prospect of her children's unhappiness. It was Claudia's own anxiety, rooted in her childhood vow to be a more nurturing parent than her own mother or father had been, that prompted her to mount preemptive indulgences toward her children: "If I cook special meals, then they won't have to eat food they don't like. If I talk to the teacher, then they won't have the burden of doing it themselves. If I just step in and smooth their way, then they won't have to face the obstacles to happiness that I faced."

Lest you attribute Claudia's anxiety to a need to be liked by her children, I can assure you that that was not the case. There was one area in which Claudia demanded a lot of her children, and that was academics. There were more than a few incidents when the kids were denied privileges because their report cards didn't have enough As, and their tearful entreaties did not sway her. When it came to doing well in school, it was as if Claudia had no anxiety whatsoever about imposing disciplinary measures on her kids. If anything, she was even more anxious about their being less-than-perfect students.

Now, years later, Claudia says that she regrets sheltering her children as much as she did and sees that they are now adults struggling with battles their peers learned to fight years ago. Gregory can't work up the courage to ask for a raise, Samantha has trouble holding on to a job because she's unwilling to do more than the minimum required by her job description, and Connor is still in college after six years because he can't decide what he wants to do with his life and keeps changing his major. Gregory, Samantha, and Connor are all very likable people; they are intelligent and congenial and treat their friends and parents with kindness and respect. But they are also unable to tolerate more than the most minor discomfiture; they are thrown into emotional disarray when faced with disappointment and lack the resilience that enables more competent adults to bounce back after a major upset.

Which is a hazard of having a primitive-preventive relationship with your anxiety: in dealing with your own anxiety problem, you may create problems for the very people you're trying to protect.

BERNICE: "I CAN'T BEAR THE THOUGHT OF ONE OF THEM HAVING SOMETHING THE OTHER ONE DOESN'T"

Consider Bernice, the mother of eighteen-year-old identical twin girls. Bernice said she had always been a bit on the anxious side but now found she was unable to turn the anxiety off. She was having stomach problems and difficulty sleeping, and she complained that she had aged a decade in just a few months. She mentioned having competed in beauty pageants when she was younger, and said that she'd always been able to get back to a normal sleep schedule once the competition was over. But now Bernice's insomnia was making her too groggy to focus on her volunteer work in the front office of the twins' school and she hoped she might get a prescription to help her sleep. Bernice said she was interested neither in long-term therapy nor in coming in for weekly sessions, but merely in getting something to help her sleep through the night. The doctor said she'd consider that once they had a chance to talk, and she asked Bernice if there was anything going on that might be boosting her anxiety level.

"Sure, there is," Bernice said. "We're waiting to hear from colleges." She sighed heavily.

"I'm sure you know from talking to other parents that it's quite typical for students to be stressed out by the application process," the doctor said.

"You don't understand; Shannon and Kiara are not your typical high school students. These girls have almost straight As since middle school; they're taking almost all AP courses—that's advanced placement—and their SATs are really good. If you haven't had kids at this level of intelligence, you don't know what it's like." Bernice shifted in her seat and sighed before continuing.

"There were all these applications to fill out and recommendations and test scores to get sent. They do a lot of it online now, and it's nerve-wracking because you don't know for sure if it all got there. And the essays they had to write! You'd think they were applying for the Nobel Prize."

"How are the girls handling the fact that they haven't heard yet?"

"Oh, they've heard, except for Hopkins. Shannon got in, but Kiara's on the waiting list. They both want to do premed, and Hopkins is their first choice. If Kiara doesn't get in it'll be terrible, just terrible."

"Has Kiara been accepted anywhere?"

Bernice looked startled. "Of course!" she said. "She's gotten in everywhere except Hopkins. But she'll be devastated if she can't go there. She and Shannon have always been together, and I don't know how Kiara will handle it if she has to go to college alone."

"What about Shannon?" the doctor said.

"Shannon? What about her?" Bernice asked.

"You just said Kiara would be devastated if she had to go to college without Shannon. Well, if Kiara doesn't get into Hopkins, wouldn't Shannon be going to college without Kiara?" Bernice thought for a moment.

"It's not the same thing," she said. "Shannon would be going to her first choice and Kiara wouldn't. You can't compare the two. It's driving me crazy. I can't concentrate at work; I get into bed at night with my stomach in knots. I never thought applying to college would be so stressful."

"How are the girls handling it?"

"The girls seem all right, but how much do you know with these kids? It's not as if Kiara's going to tell me what she's really going through. Whenever I try to talk to her, she tells me I should chill and get a life."

The doctor spoke gently: "Well, she may have a point. It sounds as if you're more invested in the Hopkins waiting list than your daughters are."

A weary look passed over Bernice's face. "When you have kids like this, you have to be invested. This isn't just about college; it's about medical school, too. Coming out of Hopkins, there's no way Shannon won't get into medical school. But what if Kiara goes somewhere that's not as prestigious? How is she going to feel if Shannon gets into medical school and she doesn't? I've been thinking of calling the admissions committee at Hopkins to see if they'll move Kiara up on the waiting list, but my husband thinks it's a bad idea. I might do it anyway."

Mothers may not have a monopoly on primitive-preventive anxiety relationships, but it's safe to say they are probably overrepresented in the category (as they are in this chapter). And though there are plenty of childless people who have this kind of relationship with some or all of their anxieties, I have chosen mothers for my depictions because the mindless, gut-level urge to promote your children's best interests and protect them from hurt are compulsions most of us can relate to.

Which brings us back to Bernice and her machinations to protect her daughters from the anguish and disappointment she imagined they would suffer were she not to smooth their way. From the time they were born, Bernice had been hyperaware of their twinness, if not their sameness: she said she had never dressed them alike, had intentionally chosen names that sounded dissimilar, and had requested that the school put them in different kindergarten classes (until someone told her that Mrs. Wade was the best teacher, so she lobbied for both Kiara and Shannon to be put in her class, and they were). Bernice began volunteering in the school office several days a week to have an inside edge on hearing about any and all developments that might be advantageous to the girls. When a full-time administrative position became available, she took the job; when the girls moved on to middle school, she began volunteering there, as she did when they moved up to high school.

Bernice kept close tabs on Kiara's and Shannon's schoolwork, collaborating with them on projects and proofreading their papers after they were asleep, inputting corrections and printing out fresh copies before the twins awoke in the morning. She said she got upset when one got a better grade than the other on an assignment and spoke at length about a science project that had earned one an A and the other a C-plus, citing the teacher's refusal to change the grade even after Bernice intervened. Bernice also spoke of her struggle when Shannon made the varsity volleyball team and Kiara didn't. Bernice met with the coach and pressed her to put both of them on the team; when the coach refused, Bernice said it had taken weeks for her stomach to calm down.

Over the course of Bernice's therapy, she revealed a consistent pattern of micromanaging her daughters' lives, all in the name of advocating for their best interests and protecting them from harm. From all appearances, the girls were fully capable of absorbing the shocks that so jolted their mother; there was no evidence that either Shannon or Kiara was devastated at the prospect of attending a different college than the other—disappointed, perhaps, but not devastated. They acknowledged being somewhat competitive with each other but evinced none of the emotional fragility their mother spoke of.

The emotional fragility, of course, dwelt within Bernice and not her daughters; it was she, not they, who was anguished at the prospect of one girl having something the other wanted and did not have. Bernice's anxiety was all about fending off the pain she felt for her daughters' sakes; the irony was that neither of them felt it nearly as acutely as she did.

Bernice's doctor prescribed an antianxiety medication, with the understanding that she would also commit to doing some stress-reducing activities. Bernice said she could commit to taking a brisk thirty-minute walk at least four times a week and also promised to restring her guitar and practice every day. Bernice returned two months later and reported that she had begun sleeping a little better and that her stomach had calmed down, and that Kiara had been admitted to Hopkins. This was a great relief to the girls, Bernice said, who had decided to room with other people but live in the same dormitory. To those of us hearing about the case, it was clear that Bernice's relief was at least as great as her daughters'.

Bernice's doctor continues to see her once every few months, typically when she feels the need to talk or her prescription needs refilling. The doctor says the medication has alleviated some of Bernice's symptoms but that her anxiety is far from gone. "Now she's anxious about the pressure the girls are facing as premeds," the doctor told me. "She's convinced that no one is looking out for them and making sure they're thriving and emotionally stable. What she doesn't seem able to understand yet is that Kiara and Shannon are doing that for themselves."

Even though Bernice and Claudia employ different measures to quell their anxiety, they provide good illustrations of people who relate to it in a primitive-preventive way. And although they are less able to tolerate their children's discomfort than most mothers I know of, I would suggest that both of them fall within the spectrum of normal. I say this because their coping strategies, however eccentric, are not utterly out of the ordinary: I know of quite a few mothers who don't require their children to partake of the main dinner entrée or go to bed at a set time; I also know of many parents who are, in my opinion, too quick to leap in and rescue their preadolescent and teenage kids from situations the kids should be handling themselves. These coping strategies are far from harmless: as we have seen, Claudia's grown children are not always confident of their ability to advocate and care for themselves; indeed, Claudia still feels compelled to rescue them when they hit a snag (as when she recently offered to fly cross-country to nurse Samantha through a particularly nasty bout of the flu; happily, Samantha declined and made it through on her own). Still, I would say that both Claudia's and Bernice's anxiety are within the normal range.

Daria, however, was another story.

DARIA: "I FEEL SO POWERLESS TO OVERCOME THIS TERROR. I'VE BEEN ALLOWING IT TO RUN MY LIFE"

Daria was thirty-two years old and worked as a buyer of women's accessories for an upscale department store when she first became my patient. She was married, the mother of a preschooler, and, from the look of it, had another child on the way. When I asked her what had brought her in to see me, she said she had a lot of anxiety and the only way she could think of dealing with it was to quit her job, only she didn't want to quit her job and didn't know what to do.

"Is the job making you anxious?" I asked.

"Oh, no—I love my job. And we need the money, especially with another baby on the way," she said.

"Okay. You love the job and you need the job. So why do you think your anxiety will lessen if you quit the job?"

Daria explained that her mother, who cared for her son, Gavin, while Daria was at work every day, was leaving for a monthlong cruise and Daria was going to have to put the three-year-old in day care. Daria said she had resisted putting Gavin in day care because she was terrified that he might get sick. I asked her if she was worried that she couldn't get time off from work to care for him or if he had health issues that might result in complications.

"No, that's not it," she said. "My husband, Tom, is also going away, on a business trip, and if Gavin gets sick and my mother's not there and Tom's not there I'll have to do everything myself and I might freak out and if I freak out I won't be able to take care of Gavin, and if I can't take care of him . . ." Daria's voice trailed off, and she looked down at her lap.

It took a while, but the story finally emerged. Daria was wracked with anxiety not because she was obsessed with germs or because she was afraid of being alone with her child or because she didn't know how to take care of him; she was suffering because she had an irrational and paralyzing fear of vomit.

Now, I've never met anyone who enjoys vomiting, or at least anyone who admits to enjoying it; vomit is one of those things that tends to inspire in most of us varying degrees of distaste. But Daria's response transcended distaste; Daria was so repulsed at the prospect of encountering vomit that she was convinced that, were her son to get sick and throw up, she would be too freaked out to clean him up and take care of him. She pictured worst-case scenarios in which her young son thrashed in his bed, feverish and soiled and crying out for her, while she cowered in the next room, unable to come to his aid. Rather than risk neglecting her child because of her fear, she had kept Gavin isolated from other children, refusing to place him in day care, declining almost all play dates, and keeping him indoors if there was any threat of inclement weather. Things had gotten so bad that she was now ready to forfeit her job and its much-needed income to avoid having to send her son to day care and expose him to other children and the germs they carried.

As you may have guessed, Daria, like my friend Merle, was suffering from a specific phobia. What qualifies both women's experience as a phobia rather than an intense yet normal response is that they both have irrational, involuntary fear reactions that are inappropriate to the situation because there is no real threat of danger. It is the irrational, involuntary nature of the anxiety that places both Daria and Merle in the abnormal range on the anxiety spectrum—that and the fact that even though they know their anxiety makes no sense, they are unable to reason their way out of it.

Daria said the first time she remembered being terrified of vomit was in seventh grade, when a boy in her math class threw up and it got all over his ruler and loose-leaf binder and his desk was covered with it and all the kids were grossed out.

"I didn't outgrow it, either," she said. "The night my husband proposed, in the midst of all my joy, I remember thinking, What if I get pregnant and get morning sickness? Even if I don't get it, what if the baby . . . ? I knew it was crazy, but that's what went through my mind when Tom proposed.

"Last week I actually wrote a letter resigning from my job, but I couldn't bring myself to sign it. This voice inside me kept shrieking, What are you doing? This isn't what you want! But I feel so powerless to overcome this terror that I've been allowing it to run my life. I simply cannot believe I'm thinking of quitting my job because I'm afraid my child will, well, you know. It's completely nuts, and I *know* it's nuts, but I still can't stop it."

But Daria did stop it. She agreed to come back once a week and embark on a program of desensitization therapy. We began slowly, talking about the dreaded act of vomiting and practicing saying the word. I then sent away to a practical joke shop for some phony pet vomit with the intention of getting Daria to be able to look at it, hold it, and perhaps even laugh at it. At the beginning of the session she could barely stand to look at it in the package, but by the end she was able to prod it with her finger. Several sessions later, we went online and watched some pretty disgusting videos of young people throwing up—gross, perhaps, but ultimately a triumphal course of therapy: Daria is no longer paralyzed by either the thought or reality of vomit, which is fortunate because not long afterward she gave birth to her second child, who for a time suffered from infant reflux. She says that although she's able to cope with the bouts of stomach flu that go around every season, she still isn't crazy about dealing with vomit. But, as I say to her, who is?

The primitive-preventive relationship is, like the other anxiety relationships, characterized by its nature, not its severity: both Claudia and Bernice, whose anxiety was within the normal range, and Merle and Daria, who suffer from phobias, relate to their anxiety in this way. If you tend to engage in behaviors or perform occasional rituals, however innocuous, to prevent an anxiety-provoking situation, you too may be relating to your anxiety in a primitive-preventive way. I grew up in New York, where we had wide, cracked sidewalks. We used to chant, "Step on a crack, break your mother's back," and I'd think, Gee, maybe I shouldn't take a chance, so I'd avoid the cracks. Or when people see a black cat coming toward them, many think, Aw, I think I'll cross the street.

Then there are those mythical dos and don'ts that are passed down from one generation to the next. A superstition in my family is that you should never buy or rent a green car. My grandmother told me this when I was a little girl, and when I asked my father about it he said, "That's right, we'd never have a green car. I don't know why, but your grandma always told me not to do it." I went back to my grandmother, but she couldn't tell me how it had started, either. Even so, whenever I've gone to rent a car, I've heard myself saying, "Can you please make sure it's not a green one?" (Of course, I'd never *buy* a green car, either.) It's not an obsession, and it's not a phobia; I don't even know what sort of dread occurrence I'm trying to prevent. Still, I feel more comfortable if I stay away from green cars. Irrational? Yes. Eccentric? Perhaps. Primitive-preventive? Absolutely.

MIGHT I HAVE A PRIMITIVE-PREVENTIVE RELATIONSHIP WITH MY ANXIETY?

1. Do you routinely take action to protect yourself from anxiety before analyzing the consequences of the action?
2. Do you (or people close to you) think you react too quickly and thoughtlessly to stressful situations?
3. Do you find yourself manipulating people and situations to prevent yourself from feeling anxious?
4. Do you feel driven by a need to protect your loved ones from situations, events, and people who do not pose any actual, inherent danger to them?
5. Do you feel compelled to perform unnecessary behaviors and rituals that you believe may somehow protect your loved ones from danger?

seven

THE IMPERATIVE-FUGITIVE RELATIONSHIP

Imperative: an unavoidable fact compelling or insistently calling for action

Fugitive: running away or intending flight

Two months into my own treatment for breast cancer, I got a call from my surgeon, asking if I would help a woman who had come to see her. The woman had a phobia about medical procedures that was preventing her from getting a biopsy of what felt to the doctor like a large and possibly cancerous lump. My immediate response was "Absolutely—have her call me, and I'll fit her in right away."

I met Phyllis in my office that evening. I'm pretty good at judging people's ages, but Phyllis was hard to read. Dressed in a voluminous black sweater that concealed the contours of her body, she might have been anywhere from forty to fifty-five; her smooth complexion gave nothing away, nor did her long hair, which she wore in dreadlocks barely touched by gray.

6. Are you preoccupied with or distracted by thoughts of harm befalling you or your loved ones and what you must do to prevent it from happening, even when you recognize that these thoughts are irrational?
7. Does this relationship work for you?
   a. Positive aspects:

   b. Negative aspects:

"I don't know why I'm here," she said. "The only reason I came is because the doctor said you were used to people like me and that you'd been through this whole thing yourself. I just don't see how I can go through with it. And if I don't, I'm going to die." Her face crumpled, and the tears began to flow.

Phyllis said she was divorced, lived alone, and worked as a conservator at a folk art museum. Childless by choice, she had minimal contact with her parents and siblings, whom she described as disapproving of her lifestyle—"They drifted away when they realized I was never going to remarry and have kids, as was expected of me," she said. To compensate, she had developed an extended network of friends, but even they were keeping their distance because they were frustrated with her refusal to seek medical care. My heart went out to her.

Phyllis said she had first felt the lump nearly a year before and had finally gone to her internist because she had begun to fear for her life. He had referred her to the surgeon, and when she told Phyllis that it was imperative that she have a biopsy right away, Phyllis had refused, saying she was terrified of needles: she hadn't gone near a needle since she was a kid, and said she would rather let the cancer kill her than get an injection. But she was equally frightened of the disease and devastated that she had allowed her anxiety to possibly jeopardize her life. She sat in my office sobbing and repeating, "I just can't do it, I just can't do it." I think she cried for the entire hour the first time she came in.

Every once in a while a patient walks into your office and you realize that you have been given the sacred opportunity to change the outcome of her life. For me, Phyllis was one of those patients. And as it happens, she had perhaps the most dramatic imperative-fugitive anxiety relationship I have ever seen: so profound was her fear, she was willing to pay almost any price to evade it. Talk about a life-and-death scenario; this was it. There was no point in telling Phyllis she might die if the tumor turned out to be malignant; she knew that. Nor was there any point in telling her that the discomfort or pain of a biopsy—or even surgery—was minor compared to the consequences of doing nothing; she knew that as well. Phyllis's intelligence and common sense were useless to her; all she knew was that she might die unless she overcame her fear of needles, and she just couldn't imagine doing it.

I enjoy the challenge of complicated cases and knew that if anyone could help Phyllis, I could. I thought back to the woman I'd worked with who hadn't left her apartment in more than thirty years. For my first session with Grace, I went to her home and managed to get her not only out the front door but to touch the windshield of my car, which was parked in front of her building.* If you can imagine what it must feel like to lock the door of your apartment when gasoline costs eighteen cents a gallon and not emerge again until *Annie Hall* wins the Oscar for best picture—and I'm not sure anyone can—you'll get an idea of the disorientation and terror Grace must have felt as she ventured out that day. Yet she did it. And not only that: as we worked together over the next five months, Grace enrolled in a university program for mature learners, drove with me to Baltimore to appear on a local television show (cohosted by an extraordinary new talent, Oprah Winfrey), and was taking public transportation to her part-time clerical job in a social services agency. And that was nearly twenty-five years in the past. If I was able to help Grace and others like her overcome their disabling fears, I knew I could help Phyllis.

However, working with Phyllis turned out to be challenging in ways I hadn't anticipated. When you go through a fearsome experience, it's common to become acutely sensitive to information relating to what you have been through, which was very much the case with me. During my illness, I was as passionate about seeking information and as comforted by acquiring it as I ever was. But when Phyllis became my patient, I lost control both over how and when I got information about breast cancer, which

* You can read more about Grace in my first book, *Triumph Over Fear.*

turned out to be deeply unsettling. As it turned out, Phyllis was as energetic an information seeker as I was and would sometimes bring me news that would distract me from the matter at hand, which was to help her with her problem, not think about my own. If she spoke of a new treatment she had just read about, my mind would start racing: Does my doctor know about this? Remember to mention it at my next visit. And after she came in one day with news about just-announced side effects of a popular cancer drug, I found myself worrying that she would come in next time and tell me that they'd just discovered that one of the medications I was taking would actually cause something that was far worse than what I already had.

Emotionally, it was the perfect storm: there I was, talking to a woman who might have a life-threatening disease and who was not going for treatment. I understood intellectually that Phyllis's phobia was as real as it was irrational, and had she been capable of managing it, she wouldn't be in my office. But on an emotional level, it was wrenching for me to hear her say that she'd rather die than get an injection when I myself was willing to do whatever it took to get well. My feelings ran the gamut: sometimes I wanted to tell her, "Just do it!" as I had so often heard my patients' family members exhort them to just overcome their phobias, which I knew was completely preposterous; other times I wanted to put my arms around her and comfort her as she cried. Most of all, I felt a powerful urge to rescue this woman from the clutches of death, and I found myself thinking about things I might do to prevent her from suffering the anguish of being sick, frightened, and alone. It was as though I were facing a deeply troubled, less fortunate version of myself, and it gave me pause: What might my life be like without a devoted husband and family to help me through my illness? How would I have approached treatment were my phobia about needles rather than heights? Indeed, what would my life be like had I never sought treatment for my phobia, as Phyllis had never sought treatment for hers? Why was I strong enough, trained enough, fortunate enough, insured enough, whatever enough to be treated for this disease when Phyllis and so many other women were not?

I began to realize that I was not able to do for this patient what I was able to do for others, what was indeed my obligation to do as a clinician: to distance myself from my own feelings enough to be sufficiently objective to help her with hers. As a therapist, I knew it was absolutely necessary to maintain boundaries between my patients and myself; otherwise, my innermost thoughts and feelings would become entangled with those of the patient and the relationship would shift from professional to personal. I felt Phyllis deserved every break she could get and that it was my obligation to empower her to save her own life. I also knew that I would have trouble maintaining the boundaries separating us because there was so much about her situation that resonated with my own. I realized, finally, that I was still too raw and vulnerable to fulfill my obligations to this patient.

With this in mind, I decided to do for Phyllis what I typically do when a new patient comes in with a medical phobia: I referred her to Judy, a nurse who has worked with me for almost thirty years and has a gift for dealing with all sorts of phobias, particularly those relating to doctors, hospitals, needles, and the like. Not only was (and is) Judy knowledgeable about medical procedures, she routinely accompanies patients into medical offices, dental offices, and even delivery rooms to help them confront their fears. There was no doubt in my mind that Judy was the ideal person to work with Phyllis.

Phyllis was initially apprehensive about switching therapists but adapted remarkably well. In fact, after working with Judy, Phyllis was able to undergo a biopsy, surgery to remove the tumor, and a regimen of chemotherapy. As much as I wanted to treat Phyllis myself, I knew this was the right decision both for her and for me. After some time had passed, I began to see that the anxiety I experienced during my sessions with Phyllis was primitive-preventive in nature: the primitive anxiety I felt about needing to save her life—as well as my own—conflicted with my need to prevent an onslaught of information from diverting my attention away from her situation and onto my own. As I sat in session with Phyllis and heard about this new study or that just-discovered (and harmful) side effect, I experienced an inner turmoil I was professionally bound to hide. Even though Phyllis had only two or three sessions with me, they were enough to prompt me to take preventive action and refer her to another therapist.

Which illustrates the benefits of recognizing how you relate to your anxiety. I didn't recognize it with utter clarity at the time, of course; all I knew was that the surgeon who had saved my life had called and asked if I could help her save someone else's. But when I finally did recognize and understand that my own primal life-and-death anxiety was the source of my inner tumult, I was able to do not only what was right for my patient but also what was right for me.

Phyllis is, of course, someone whose anxiety falls well outside the normal range. But I chose to open the chapter with her because the sheer extremity of her anxiousness provides an unambiguous illustration of the imperative-fugitive relationship. The words that capture this relationship most aptly in its normal-range manifestations are "I'd rather die," as in "Stand up and propose a toast in front of three hundred people? I'd rather die" or "Go out in a bathing suit with *these* thighs? I'd rather die" or "Ride a roller coaster that flips you upside down? I'd rather die." No matter how much you dread speaking in front of a roomful of gowned and tuxedoed wedding guests, baring your middle-aged flesh to a bunch of strangers at the beach, or subjecting yourself to G-force physical abuse that scores of daredevils are waiting in line to experience, chances are that, actually pressed, you probably would rather endure the concomitant humiliations, indignities, and terrors than relinquish your life. Which is to say that when normal-spectrum anxious folks say they would rather die than endure the intense anxiety and discomfort brought on by participating in a dreaded activity, they mean it figuratively; when abnormal-spectrum folks like Phyllis say they would rather die than do something, they may mean it literally, or at least think they do. When Phyllis said she would rather die of cancer than have an injection, she did not mean it 100 percent literally; if she had, she would not have been in my office. Still, her paralyzing anxiety disabled her from thinking rationally and made her feel as if death were her only option.

The predominant sensation associated with the imperative-fugitive relationship is an urge to run, escape, or hide from anxious feelings when they start to arise. You might say it's characterized by a flight, *not* fight, response; if you have an imperative-fugitive relationship with your anxiety—and many if not most of us have it with at least some of our anxieties—you are familiar with that inner voice shrieking "Aaaaargh! Go! Go! Go! Get out of here now!" It's that feeling you get when you've just steered your shopping cart into the produce aisle and see that horrid person you argued with several days earlier, and before you know it you're burning rubber en route to the dairy case. Or when a guy at work asks you out for Saturday night but you'd much rather go to a party you've been invited to, so you make up a story about going out of town for the weekend and then he shows up at the party, just like that, and you start looking for a window to escape through. Or when an attentive saleswoman spends an hour and a half bringing you tops, bottoms, camisoles, and coordinating jackets until you put together the perfect outfit, which, when you get home, turns out to be not so perfect after all, and you go to return it but keep skulking away because every time you show up she's there behind the counter and you're too embarrassed to face her.

The situations that transform us into fugitives from anxiety aren't limited to face-to-face confrontations, of course; many common ones tend to involve a commitment of one kind or another. For example, most of us know at least one couple who have been living together forever and say they intend to get married but who just can't manage to do the deed; there's always a pressing concern that postpones the idea of legalizing the partnership. (I'm not talking about couples who prefer to live together without being married but about couples who allegedly aspire to the wedded state.) I have no scientific data on this but would wager that most of the time, the delays are diversionary tactics obscuring the fact that either one or both of the persons involved feel anxious about publicly formalizing the commitment, whether they know it or not.

A commitment need not be romantic to inspire evasive maneuvers. I once treated a very nice guy who came in for help with a phobia about driving over bridges. He was in his forties, had a wife and three children, and worked in the accounting department of a music publisher. One day he came in as happy as could be and told me that he and his wife had found their dream house. They had been renting an apartment and looking for a bigger place, he said, and had finally found a four-bedroom, all-brick colonial in an established neighborhood that was zoned for the school district they wanted. They had put down a deposit and planned to move in several months' time, after the school year ended.

Time passed, and I asked my patient how the move was coming along. He said things were progressing slowly because he kept missing paperwork deadlines, which he said was odd, given his conscientious nature. He kept forgetting to schedule the inspection of the new place and was procrastinating about calling lenders to secure a mortgage. His wife was getting annoyed; she was running around doing all the legwork because he couldn't seem to manage it, and moreover, she was becoming anxious that they wouldn't be ready to close on time. In the end, the deal fell through. My patient lost his $22,000 deposit, roughly equivalent to $50,000 today.

"I'm forty-three, and we have three kids to put through school," he said. "I'd still be paying for that house well into my seventies! What if we didn't have enough money for college? Or new cars, or the doctor, or food?" Granted, borrowing a six-figure sum and signing a thirty-year mortgage is a sobering rite of passage, as well it should be: a house is the biggest investment most of us ever make. But it is also the safest one, according to most financial experts, and the bottom line is that in addition to his fear of driving over bridges, this man had intense anxiety about money. By evading the procedures required to complete the sale, he successfully fled the anxiety associated with a hefty financial commitment. (He also angered his wife in the process, but that's another story.)

The imperative-fugitive relationship is also frequently seen in the context of fear of success. I know a stay-at-home mother in her late thirties who studied metallurgy in college and creates striking brooches, pendants, and earrings by setting semiprecious stones in gold. Her pieces inspire fierce bidding when auctioned off at her children's schools' fund-raisers, and whenever she wears something she has made, people compliment her on it and ask where they can buy her work. A few years ago she began attending the annual gem show in Tucson—a big event for anyone involved in the jewelry trade—and she comes home every year with a fistful of business cards from store owners and online vendors interested in selling her work. Yet she has never followed up on a single contact.

"It's not that I think I do substandard work. It's just that when I think about showing my work to real professionals, I get nervous that they'll realize my pieces aren't as good as they looked when they saw me wearing them," she says. There's nothing extraordinary about this; most of us would feel at least a twinge of anxiety at the prospect of our fledgling creations being evaluated by experts. What is extraordinary is this woman's willingness to allow her anxiety to quash numerous legitimate opportunities to build her avocation into a viable business. As I see it, she's not anxious about people seeing her pieces as long as they understand that they were created by a homemaker: in her mind, no one would expect a stay-at-home mom to be capable of professional-level work, nor would anyone belittle her for being mediocre at a hobby. But the moment she imagines portraying herself as a professional metalsmith, she's beset by anxiety that her work won't live up to professional standards. Any encouragement she might feel at the gem show is consistently overwhelmed by anxiety that she'll be exposed as mediocre, and her incipient career remains stalled.

If running from anxiety can cause a new career to stall, it can also cause an established career to founder. Consider a scenario I mentioned a few chapters ago, that of the executive who sent protégés on speaking assignments because she was too anxious to do them herself. This example was provided in the context of a pervasive-adaptive relationship, in which the executive adapted to her anxiety by routinely having her subordinates carry out the dreaded activity in her stead. The outcome was not entirely negative: the junior staff got experience, and the senior person was spared a series of distressing ordeals.

But in the context of an imperative-fugitive relationship, the outcome could be quite different. I once treated a midlevel manager who came in after a crisis at work. For years Olivia had camouflaged her fear of public speaking under the cover of family commitments. The mother of four children, she had bowed out of several speaking engagements because her presence was allegedly required at her children's athletic practices, music recitals, and teacher conferences. Olivia made much of the importance of balancing work and family life and won the approbation of the young people on her staff, who were more than happy to substitute for her when she was called upon to speak. But one day she was called upon at a staff meeting to get up and give an impromptu report. As she described it, she lurched to the front of the room as if she were inebriated; the place was spinning, she couldn't focus on what she wanted to say, and by the time she sat down her blouse was so drenched with perspiration she felt as if someone had poured a bucket of water over her.

Olivia felt humiliated in front of her colleagues and fell into a depression punctuated by piercing anxiety about her professional future, which was when she decided to seek help. The good news is that we were able to desensitize Olivia to her public speaking anxiety, and in time she was able to take on some speaking assignments, although not all; she still delegates a few to her subordinates. Which is fine: you don't have to subject yourself to every crazy-making circumstance just to prove you're no longer running away from your anxiety. If you think you may be forcing yourself to face anxiety-provoking situations just to prove something, ask yourself: "If this situation [encounter, experience] didn't make me anxious, would I still be doing it?" If the answer is no, don't do it. If the answer is yes, then do it and deal with the anxiety.

For example, imagine that entertaining people in your home makes you nervous and you've been working hard to overcome the anxiety. You've had several small dinner parties for friends and even invited your husband's business partner and his wife over for cocktails. Then your husband asks if it's okay for him to invite his ex-wife, from whom he divorced amicably, and her husband to dinner. Before answering him, ask yourself: "If I didn't have a problem with entertaining, would I invite my husband's ex-wife and her husband over for dinner?" If the answer is yes, then go ahead and invite them, even if it makes you anxious. On the other hand if the answer is "No way—she's never been civil to me, and I don't want her in my home," then tell your husband, honestly, that you don't want to invite his ex-wife to dinner because of how she behaves toward you. Don't blame your anxiety. Yes, you should practice facing your fears, but you also should give yourself permission not to do something you don't want to do if you're doing it just to prove you can.

HOLLY: "SOME PEOPLE OUT THERE ACTUALLY WENT TO ART SCHOOL. HOW CAN I COMPETE WITH THEM?"

No one could accuse Holly of overreaching. After four years at a competitive state university, from which she graduated cum laude with a major in art and a minor in English, the one thing she felt qualified to do was froth milk all day in pursuit of the perfect latte. Which is exactly what she was doing—that and all manner of steam-propelled, coffee-related processes and procedures—in her part-time job as a barista in an upscale neighborhood coffeehouse. Holly hadn't been working there that long; it was only seven months since graduation. And it wasn't that bad: the work was hard, but she was there only part-time, and the employees were okay and the customers mostly pleasant.

"It's not forever; it's just until I figure out . . . you know, until I get a job in my field," she said at her first session with her therapist.

Holly's field was graphic design, and she knew that she had to create a résumé and start going on interviews. But whenever she started to put her history down on paper, she became discouraged and quit.

"It's not as if I've done anything," she said. "My senior project won a prize, so I guess that's something. But that's, like, so nothing compared to what some people out there have done. Kids who go to art school win prizes all the time. How can I compete with them? Why would anyone want to hire me when they can have someone who went to Parsons or Otis or SCAD?"

"Scad?" the therapist said.

"Savannah College of Art and Design. It's a great place. My friend Rebecca went there, and she got a job at an advertising agency, like, before she even graduated. Kids coming out of there really know what they're doing. It's not like I can compete with that."

In fact, Holly didn't feel she could compete at all. Like the stay-at-home mother whose anxiety prevented her from seeing herself as a professional metalsmith, Holly's anxiety prevented her from seeing herself as a professional, period. She had been able to interview for and get the barista job because she had been brewing and drinking coffee for years and didn't think of slinging caffeine as a profession. But the thought of creating a résumé, sending out letters, and trying to get interviews as a graphic designer filled her with dread, as it does so many young people when they're just starting out.

Holly's anxiety went beyond the fear of rejection and concomitant procrastination associated with making cold calls. One day she said she had gotten an email from Rebecca saying her agency was hiring designers and that she'd chatted up Holly to the art director, who had agreed to talk to her. Rebecca had provided his name and email address and told Holly to contact him right away because those positions tended to go fast.

"What are you going to do?" the therapist asked. Holly looked glum.

"It's too late," Holly said. "They hired someone else." It turned out that Holly had waited four days before emailing the art director. By that time, he had interviewed seven people, chosen two finalists, and offered the job to one of them. He didn't feel he needed to see anyone else.

Holly wasn't just avoiding making opportunities for herself; she was fleeing opportunities others were making for her. This wasn't a cold-calling situation but rather one in which she had had the equivalent of a letter of introduction. Her anxiety was such that even when she was halfway in the door, the feelings were still strong enough to pull her back out. What could make an honors graduate of a good school so anxious about competing in the real world?

Information about Holly's family life provided some clues. She lived at home with her parents and younger brother. Her older brother, Ian, an assistant district attorney in New York City, had graduated from Columbia Law School and passed the New York bar exam on his first try. Holly said Ian had always been the one her parents favored, the child they always figured would make it in the professional world. Zach, her younger brother, was finishing his associate's degree at a local college and commuted to class. Although he had never distinguished himself academically,

Holly's parents had always emphasized the importance of his and Ian's education over hers.

"My mother dropped out of college to marry my father, and I don't think she ever got over it," Holly said. "Between the two of them, she's the one with the energy and the drive, only it's focused on the house and her kids and all these little projects she gets involved in. She's frustrated and angry but she won't admit it, and she uses her disappointments to defend her own bad choices. It's, like, just because she didn't finish college, I should be grateful that I was allowed to go at all. Ian went to Cornell undergrad and Columbia Law, and they would have sent Zach to private school if he'd been able to get in. But even though I graduated in the top ten percent of my class I was only allowed to apply to state schools, nothing private. All I ever heard was 'It's more important for a boy to go to a top school because he'll have to support a family someday. A girl will be supported by her husband.' That's my dad's line. Meanwhile, Ian's wife works for a Park Avenue law firm and makes more than he does, but I never hear Dad say anything about that."

Holly knew that her parents' attitudes about education were backward, and she had no trouble expressing her resentment about it. But years of indoctrination had eroded her confidence and left her too weak to assert herself. Living at home wasn't helping, either. Holly's mother was contemptuous of the job she had taken—"Why didn't you tell us you wanted to run around making coffee all day—oh, I mean part of the day? We could have saved a truckload of money on tuition"—and Zach openly disparaged Holly's willingness to take the abuse.

"He puts me down constantly for not telling Mom to buzz off, but how can I do that? I'm living in her house, eating her food, and watching her HBO. I can't afford to move out on a part-time salary. I've got to get a real job, but I don't know how I can do that. The thought of going in for an interview and sitting there and trying to convince them to hire me—forget it. I'd rather die."

Holly's assertion that she would rather die than go on an interview was, of course, not meant literally. But even though her situation was not as dramatic as Phyllis's, her anxiety was equally indicative of an imperative-fugitive relationship: to Holly, avoiding interviewing for meaningful work felt just as necessary as avoiding needles felt to Phyllis. The essence of the relationship lies in its effects, not its drama, and, were Holly's anxiety allowed to fester, she might still be living at home twenty years hence and quite possibly be depressed as well.

The therapist decided to approach the case by getting Holly to think concretely about what she was feeling.

"Holly, what is it that frightens you so much about going on interviews?"

"I'm not frightened of interviews," she said. "I actually enjoy talking to people."

"Good. So tell me what you think will happen when you go on an interview."

"Well, they'll read my résumé and ask me questions and I'll have to answer them."

"And then what will happen?"

"Well, I might not be able to answer the questions. Or maybe I will."

"And then what will happen?"

"I guess I'll either get the job, or I won't."

"Let's say you don't get the job. What would happen next?" Holly shifted in her seat.

"I'd feel embarrassed. And I'd know I was going to have to go through the whole thing all over again someplace else."

"So that's what might happen if you don't get the job. Now, let's say you do get the job. What would happen then?"

"Whoa! I've never gotten that far, even in my imagination."

"Try to imagine it now. What do you think will happen if you get the job?"

"If I get the job they'll give me all these things to do, and I might not know how to do them and it'll be a total disaster."

"Let's stay with that thought a moment," the therapist said. "It's your first day on the job and they show you your office and give you an assignment and you don't know what to do. What's the worst thing that could happen?" Holly studied a box of tissues on the table before answering.

"I'd have to ask somebody to show me how to do it."

"Okay. So you ask someone to show you. Then what?"

"I'm sure they'd help me. But what if I still don't understand what I have to do? I'd feel like an idiot, totally embarrassed."

"Okay. So you might not be able to do the job and you're feeling idiotic and embarrassed. Then what?"

"Well, they'd probably realize they made a mistake and they'd—"

"And they'd what? Fire you?"

"They might."

"Why would they fire you?"

"If I couldn't do the job, why would they want to keep me?"

"So what you're saying is that if you're not able to master everything your first day on the job, they'll fire you. Is that correct?"

"I guess that sounds a bit extreme. Maybe they'd give me a few more chances."

"And then what?"

"Well, the longer I'm on the job, the more they'll expect of me."

"And then what?"

"And the more they expect of me, the more I could screw up. On the first day or two they'd probably have some compassion, but then they'd expect me to get it right."

"Is there any reason you wouldn't get it right?"

"I don't think so. I mean, not really, no. I was pretty good at grasping new information in school. As a matter of fact, there were some people who would always come to me for help when we got a new assignment."

"So how much of your anxiety is based in reality and how much is based on unsubstantiated negative thinking?"

"At this point, I guess it's all based on negative thinking." Holly looked sheepish. "I think I see where you're going with this."

"Another way to approach it is to ask yourself, 'What is the *possibility* that I'll mess up on the job compared to the *probability* that I'll mess up on the job?' In other words, is it possible that you'll mess up?"

"Sure, it's possible. But I don't really think it's probable because I've always been a quick learner and conscientious student." Another silence; then Holly spoke again. "Okay. I get it. I've been thinking that I'm nervous about screwing up the interview when what I'm really nervous about is screwing up the job. I'm not worried I won't get the job; I'm actually worried that I *will* get the job and that I'll be lousy at it. But I don't have any real reason to even think that."

The little "And then what?" exercise helped Holly understand that her anxiety was based in her imagination—home of "what if?" catastrophic thoughts—rather than in the reality of her solid performance in college and elsewhere. She was then able to use the exercise to challenge herself when she hit what she called the wall of her anxiety.

Once Holly understood that her fear of performing on the job was preventing her from seeking a job she really wanted, she gained insight into a fundamental component of her anxiety: taking responsibility for herself and functioning as an adult among other adults. This is a common affliction among young people entering the professional arena for the first time: for most if not all of their twenty-something years, their way has been smoothed and paid for by their parents. They're So-and-So's daughter or son, their characters, most of their beliefs, and many of their opinions forged in their parents' households. They have had limited opportunities to work with adults whose role is not to nurture, teach, or mentor them and are unaccustomed to not having allowances made for their naïveté and inexperience. Then, suddenly, they're hurled into the world of work to fend for themselves among battalions of (mostly) skilled adults wise in the ways of office practices, procedures, and politics. It's enough to make anyone anxious, even if she or he was reared in a nurturing environment.

Holly's family dynamic was less than nurturing, however. Her mother's and brother's disparaging comments, her father's passivity, and their mutual favoring of their male offspring hadn't done much for Holly's self-confidence. The fact that she was capable of producing prizewinning work had undoubtedly buoyed her up for a time, but the routine discouragement she endured at home had eroded whatever benefits the honor had conferred. And so she was mired in self-doubt and unable to get unstuck.

The turning point came when the therapist asked Holly repeatedly what the worst thing was that could happen next. This is one of my favorite therapeutic techniques, and I use it often with patients who suffer from panic attacks. Such patients are typically anxious about the consequences of having another attack, during which anxiety often manifests itself as catastrophic thinking in which the subsequent attack spirals wildly and disastrously out of control. The "What's the worst that could happen?" question sequence is particularly effective for getting these patients to see the exaggerated nature of their fears.

Here's an example of this exercise completed by Stan, a gentle thirty-seven-year-old married father of two whom I treated for panic disorder:

The worst that could happen to me during a panic attack is: *I'll lose control and go crazy.*

And then *I'll start running around wildly, flailing my arms and legs;*

And then *My wife and kids will get scared and try to stop me;*

And then *They won't be able to stop me so they'll call 911;*

And then *The cops will come and cart me off to a mental hospital;*

And then *They'll lock me in a ward and not let anybody visit me;*

And then *I'll humiliate my family and never be able to see them again;*

And then *My wife and kids won't be able to take care of themselves;*

And then *Horrible things will happen to my family—they'll starve, go unclothed;*

And then *I'll die in the hospital, and my family won't know about it;*

And then *I guess my thinking is pretty extreme; I have myself going from a panic attack to abandoning my family and dying alone in a hospital.*

Even if you don't suffer from panic disorder, you can probably relate to this line of (irrational) reasoning. It's the logic that got me planning my husband's eulogy when he was undergoing routine gallbladder surgery, and it's probably stowed somewhere in your anxiety arsenal as well, especially if you have an imperative-fugitive relationship with some (if not all) of your anxieties. If this is the case, you might want to try the "What's the worst that could happen?" exercise, a template of which can be found on page 213. If you proceed through the exercise without quitting, you will usually find that your urge to flee was motivated by a highly unrealistic, long-range view of where the anxiety might lead. When this view distorts your perspective, it is vital that you challenge its validity so you can channel your thinking in a more realistic direction.

That's what Holly's therapist was trying to get her to do. By coming to the realization that she was more afraid of botching the job than not getting it, Holly also understood that she did indeed believe she had what it took to win the job in the first place. What she had to work on was the anxiety that she would not be able to perform adequately once she was hired. In time, she was able to create a résumé, go out on interviews, and eventually secure an entry-level position at a firm in New York City. This had the added advantage of requiring her to move out of her parents' house, which went a long way toward halting the erosion of her self-confidence.

Holly's reversal of fortune resulted from a combination of willingness to explore and confront her fear and her therapist's encouragement and support while she did it. Had she not sought help to extricate herself from her anxiety, she might never have gotten beyond the belief that she wasn't good enough to succeed.

CLAIRE: "I LOST ALL MY CONFIDENCE. I NEVER DROVE AGAIN"

That's what happened to Claire, a retired New York City schoolteacher. One Sunday, as a newlywed twenty-six-year-old, she persuaded her husband to let her drive to the home of cousins they were to visit on Long Island. She was a new driver and wanted to practice on the Long Island Expressway because more and more of their relatives were moving out to the suburbs and it would be useful for her to be able to get there on her own. As Claire tells it, she pulled out of the parking spot and drove from their apartment in Queens all the way to Great Neck. Once they were off the expressway she made a right turn and, mistaking the gas pedal for the brake, accelerated when she meant to slow down and sent the car skidding onto a patch of grass. Claire jammed on the brakes and stopped the car before it hit anything, but the shock of the experience left her shaking.

"It was over sixty years ago, but I remember it as clearly as if it happened last week," Claire said recently. "The car was a big beige Chrysler. A policeman happened to see the whole thing, and he walked over. He was very friendly, said there was no harm done and that we could go on our way. But I just sat there and told him, 'I'm never driving again.' He was such a nice man; he leaned through the window and he said, 'Aw, come on, lady, nothing happened. Just start the car and continue on your way.' But that was it for me. I sat there crying for a while, and then I got out, walked around to the passenger side, and Ben got in the driver's seat.

"It wasn't like I was completely incompetent—I passed the road test on my first try. And I didn't hit anything—I remember there was a tree there and I stopped before I hit it. But I was so frightened of not driving well, of making a mistake and causing an accident, that I didn't want to take a chance. I lost all my confidence. I renewed my driver's license every four years until recently because I thought maybe someday I'd get my confidence back. But I never did. I never drove again."

Lest you picture Claire as a shy, reticent type who tends to give up easily, let me assure you that she is not. A 1941 graduate of Hunter College, she is the daughter of Russian immigrants and worked for the Navy Department during World War II. She got a college education when few women did, taught elementary school for twenty years, raised three children (including a set of twins) while working full-time, and is known for speaking her mind. She is fiercely independent and, at the age of eighty-nine, lives alone in her New York apartment (her husband died in 1992) and does everything for herself. She is afraid of no one and does not hesitate to speak her own truth to whatever power stands in the way of what she thinks is right. Yet she allowed a single automotive mishap to catalyze a formidable anxiety about driving that would last the rest of her life.

Did Claire's driving anxiety curtail her existence? Not as much as you might think. She has lived all her life in New York City and close to public transportation, which she used to commute to and from work and everywhere else she needed to go. As long-term anxieties go, Claire's has limited her life less significantly than would, say, an anxiety about using the subway. That said, she was never able to transport her children anywhere or share the driving with her husband on long family trips. And now, after years of claiming she didn't like the suburbs, she admits that part of the reason the family never moved to Long Island was that she had to live near public transportation.

If Claire's driving anxiety is a clear-cut example of an imperative-fugitive relationship, Claire herself is an example of how one person can deal with her anxieties in different ways. Claire asserts that her refusal to drive is utterly contrary to the rest of her personality, and those who know her agree. Yet the anxiety has persisted for more than sixty years because of the unique relationship Claire has with it, a relationship she has with virtually none of her other anxieties. For whatever reason, her driving anxiety is the one thing she chose to flee rather than fight, and its longevity is proof that these things don't simply diminish with time. If you have an imperative-fugitive relationship with your anxiety, you may find, as Claire did, that it's a relationship you might have for life—unless, of course, you choose to do something about it.

MIGHT I HAVE AN IMPERATIVE-FUGITIVE RELATIONSHIP WITH MY ANXIETY?

1. Do you frequently feel an urge to run, escape, or hide from common, everyday situations?
2. Are there things you need to do but avoid doing out of fear?
3. Are there things you want to do but avoid doing out of fear?
4. Are there situations you repeatedly avoid even though the avoidance may have negative consequences?
5. Does avoiding anxiety-provoking situations harm your health, career, and/or personal relationships?
6. Do friends, colleagues, and/or family members get frustrated with you because of your avoidance behaviors?

7. Is your fear of certain situations so strong that you are willing to go to extremes to avoid them?
8. Does this relationship work for you?
    a. Positive aspects:

    b. Negative aspects:

part three

MAKING IT BETTER: THE ROSS PRESCRIPTION

GETTING STARTED

By now you probably have a better understanding of your relationship—or relationship*s*—with anxiety. You know that anxiety doesn't just happen to you; it is a fluid, elastic force that, pushing or pulling, gently nudging or fiercely propelling, invites you to respond in any number and variety of ways.

So ask yourself: How is your relationship with your anxiety working for you? Is it alerting you to real hazards and inconveniences or alarming you about dangers that aren't actual threats? Is it imparting a measure of tranquillity to your conscious mind or coating your unconscious with a vague unease that prevents you from ever feeling at peace? Or is it a combination of the two—help and hindrance, good and bad?

Once you've asked yourself these questions and come up with some answers, you'll probably ask, "Okay—what do I do now?"

You read the next four chapters. Chapter 8 presents some of the latest research into the connections among anxiety, stress, and some common medical illnesses. And Chapters 9, 10, and 11 make up the Ross Prescription: a collection of exercises, questions, surveys, and documents you can do, answer, complete, and use to better understand and manage both your anxiety and your health.

The Ross Prescription contains many of the same tools and techniques that I give my patients to help them cope with and triumph over their fears and anxieties, both rational and irrational. What makes many of these strategies work well for anxiety disorders also makes them effective for everyday anxiety. Chapter 9, "Taking Inventory," will help you identify, measure, and evaluate your anxiety; Chapter 10, "Taking Action," offers suggestions and exercises for responding to your anxiety in a conscious, deliberate, constructive way; and Chapter 11, "Taking Charge," will equip you to advocate for yourself in interactions with health care professionals, family, colleagues, and friends.

eight

MANAGE YOUR ANXIETY, IMPROVE YOUR HEALTH

You now know that anxiety is not just in your head but is born of a dynamic process that is triggered in the brain and galvanizes the entire body. Its effects can be as innocuous as a night of tossing and turning in bed or as troublesome as recurring panic attacks. As you have seen, research shows that it's no longer enough to white-knuckle your way through weeks and months of anxiety-ridden days: if you want to protect your health, you have to find ways to diffuse and dispel the everyday anxiety that gnaws at the edges of your consciousness and diminishes your body's capacity to rest and heal itself.

In this chapter, you will read about the relationship that is emerging between anxiety and a variety of medical conditions, including cardiovascular disease, asthma, chronic pain, obesity, eating disorders, and substance abuse. My point is not to alarm you but rather to alert you to the numerous and sometimes mysterious ways that stress and anxiety can affect you. As you already know, I believe in arming oneself with every iota of information available; knowledge is power, after all, especially when it comes to the repercussions of living with anxiety: whereas it might lead to no more than a mild headache, it could also lead to something you would never expect.

Your fingers may, for example, erupt in tiny, itchy bumps the day after you learn your parents are divorcing after thirty-seven years of marriage or when your son tells you he is changing careers for the fourth time in as many years. What does this mean? Not even your dermatologist knows for sure. The outbreak could be a coincident allergic reaction to an ointment you applied to a scratch or an irritation caused by a new dishwashing detergent. But it could also be an outbreak of atopic dermatitis, an itchy skin rash that can be triggered or, more commonly, aggravated by anxiety and stress. Romanian scientists studying 240 people between two and sixty-seven years of age with atopic dermatitis concluded that stress was a significant factor in the participants' development of or continuing problem with the disorder. While some participants suffered outbreaks due to contact with irritating substances such as wool or allergens such as plant toxins, the researchers found that 45 percent of the cases were exacerbated by anxiety or stress.[1] In other words, even when a patient's rash was caused by an allergy or irritation, anxiety and stress either worsened the rash's severity or prolonged its presence. I know a woman who developed the condition in the midst of a family crisis and whose rash disappeared when she regained her emotional equilibrium. Although my evidence is not scientific but anecdotal and based entirely on this woman's description of the episode, the fact that her symptoms subsided along with her emotional upheaval and that she had not used any new products or medications prior to or during the outbreak leads me to believe that the dermatitis was probably triggered by anxiety and stress.

The notion that psychological perceptions, anxiety, stress, and other emotional forces influence the path of medical illness is steadily gaining credibility in Western medicine, which historically has been reluctant to acknowledge the interconnectedness of body and mind. But as more scientific research emerges that asserts the mind-body connection, it becomes increasingly clear that anxiety, stress, and ongoing emotional strain affect our health in myriad unknown ways.

For example, several 2007 studies suggest there is a link between unhappy marriages and heart disease. In Great Britain, researchers conducted a study of 9,011 civil servants, both men and women, most of whom were married, and found that those with strife-ridden relationships were 34 percent more likely to have had a heart attack or other cardiovascular problem during the twelve-month follow-up period than those with harmonious relationships. Roberto DeVogli, Ph.D., the lead author of the study, acknowledged earlier findings that marriage tends to be good for your health but said the new data showed that the quality of a person's close relationships, whether with a spouse, other intimate partner, or close friend, was more significant than merely having the bond.[2]

For women, the dynamics of primary and intimate relationships have significant health repercussions. In a long-term study of almost four thousand women and men in Framingham, Massachusetts, participants were asked whether they tended to speak up during marital disagreements or keep their mouths shut. You might be surprised to learn that women were more outspoken than their mates: only about a quarter of the women said they held their tongues, compared to nearly a third of the men. Now, here's where it gets even more interesting: over the ten years the study was in force, men who kept their feelings to themselves didn't seem to suffer any more health problems than men who spoke up. But women who kept their feelings to themselves during a fight *were four times as likely to die over the ten-year period as women who spoke their minds.*[3] It made no difference whether a woman thought she had a happy marriage or a miserable one; what mattered was whether or not she told her partner how she felt during an argument. If she consistently kept a lid on her feelings, a behavior known as self-silencing, she was unwittingly quadrupling the odds that she would die within a decade.

Another fascinating discovery is that the long-term emotional strain of tending to a chronically ill loved one can accelerate the body's aging process. As I mentioned in Chapter 3, researchers comparing the effects of stress and anxiety on mothers with healthy children to the effects on mothers with chronically ill children found that the latter developed chromosomal fraying typical of women thirteen years older.[4] And an ongoing study at Ohio State University has shown that men and women caring for spouses and parents with Alzheimer's disease also suffer premature aging of their chromosomes, equivalent to shortening their lives by four to eight years.[5]

Then there's irritable bowel syndrome. Scientists agree that psychosocial stress—that is, pressures associated with both psychological and social factors such as age, education, friendships and intimacy, and so on—plays a significant role in the onset, persistence, and severity of the condition. And it isn't just stressed-out, high-anxiety types who are vulnerable to developing the disorder: some of the calmest, coolest, most seemingly stress-proof people have fallen prey to the depredations of IBS.

Consider Ynez, a veteran publicist whose clients include a number of actors, actresses, and television personalities. Ynez typically works twelve to fourteen hours a day, most of them on the phone, negotiating deals to get her clients on talk shows and magazine covers and out of hot water when they say or do something controversial, embarrassing, or worse. She routinely deals with celebrity meltdowns and tantrums and has a reputation for being unflappable. Yet this same woman became so anxiety-ridden when planning her wedding that she developed recurrent abdominal pain and diarrhea that were diagnosed as irritable bowel syndrome (you may recall that Leslie, the investigative reporter from Chapter 5, had a history of IBS).

"I was in my late thirties and had been on my own for years," Ynez says. "My parents had divorced and remarried, and my dream was to have both of them there with their spouses and for everyone to be cordial to everyone else, which they all seemed to think was possible. So I started talking with my mother about it, and that's when the trouble started. I wanted an outside wedding, in a garden, in May; she said her allergies would be horrible so we would have to do it indoors. I wanted a picnic-style reception in the afternoon; she wanted a sit-down dinner at night. Whatever I wanted, she objected to. It was a mess long before we got to the guest list, and when we did, it became a nightmare. This one didn't want that one to be invited, that one threatened not to come if the other one was invited—it was the most stressful experience of my life. I began to dread phoning my parents because I'd always end up in the bathroom for an hour in pain. Hardly anyone was talking about irritable bowel back then, but when I went to the doctor he said he thought I might have it and asked if I'd been under any stress lately. Boy, did he get an earful."

How could Ynez be so good at handling temperamental, high-maintenance artists and wracked with anxiety when dealing with her parents? Because she found the stress of placating hysterical celebrities challenging and even amusing, maintained a healthy perspective on the absurdity of such situations, and never allowed them to affect her personally. But trying to please her estranged and demanding parents while wanting to reassure them of her abiding love and regard (and yearning to be reassured of theirs in return) preyed upon her daughterly insecurities and threw her into emotional turmoil. The conflicts roiled not only her emotions but her insides as well, manifesting as irritable bowel syndrome.

As discussed earlier, IBS is a disturbance of the gastrointestinal tract that affects 15 to 20 percent of American adults and whose symptoms commonly include abdominal pain; cramping; flatulence (gas); diarrhea or constipation, sometimes with alternating bouts of each; mucus in the stool; and a bloated feeling in the belly. Whereas IBS can be painful and distressing, it does not cause permanent damage to the intestines. Many people with IBS are able to control its symptoms by monitoring what they eat, using over-the-counter remedies (for instance, a laxative for occasional constipation), and identifying and managing the stress in their lives. We don't yet fully understand the relationship between stress, anxiety, and IBS, although we do know that they often coexist and that anxiety triggers IBS symptoms in many people who have it.[6]

So if you're the matron of honor at your best friend's wedding and a commotion starts in your stomach and you break out in a sweat because you're afraid you'll have to make a run for it in the middle of the ceremony—does this mean you have irritable bowel syndrome? No, not at all; it just probably means you're excited and nervous and more emotional than usual on your friend's big day. But if you suffer from lower abdominal pain, bouts of diarrhea and/or constipation, and unpredictable bowel activity repeatedly and frequently over a long period of time, you might want to consult a doctor and find out if irritable bowel syndrome might be causing the problem.

SO WE ALL AGREE ON THE MIND-BODY ANGLE, RIGHT? NOT SO FAST . . .

Even in the face of mounting scientific evidence, there seems to be resistance in some quarters against acknowledging the power of the mind generally and anxiety specifically to influence physiological illness. If you wander the Internet a bit and visit some health-related sites, you may occasionally find, as I have, a reluctance to associate anxiety with illnesses such as ulcerative colitis (inflammation of the colon), whose flare-ups have been found to have a connection to anxiety,[7] and fibromyalgia. To me, the reluctance manifests not as an outright refutation of anxiety's role but as a void: the term seldom if ever appears, making the notion of an anxiety component in these conditions conspicuous by its absence.

Why should this be the case? One possibility is that many American insurance companies provide only partial coverage or refuse coverage altogether for treatments of stress-related conditions. So it's better, from the patient's point of view, to be diagnosed with a physical illness and get reimbursed for the medical bills.

Another possibility is the stigma that still surrounds anxiety- and mood-related disorders. Many people are too embarrassed to acknowledge the possibility of having an anxiety issue unless they can attribute it to a physiological problem such as a chemical imbalance, for instance, or a genetic predisposition. And the stigma transcends geographical and cultural boundaries.

We used to think that anxiety and mood-related disorders were primarily a hazard of living in highly industrialized first-world countries, but now we know otherwise. A medical clinic in Siolim, a fishing and farming village in India, now employs several workers whose sole job it is to identify and treat people with anxiety and depression. The workers are part of a program started in 2005 that trains laypeople to diagnose and treat these disorders in rural Indian communities, whose inhabitants were arriving at clinics complaining of physical ailments as well as interpersonal conflicts, financial difficulties, and unemployment, among other things. The clinic physicians, who were also seeing a great deal of alcoholism in the villagers, realized that many of their patients' physical symptoms derived from psychological and emotional problems that the patients were reluctant to discuss. Under the new program, almost every patient who arrives at the clinic completes a questionnaire that asks about both physical symptoms and emotional problems, enabling the health care workers to identify those whose problems are psychological in origin. Such patients are then sent to the health counselor, who explains what anxiety and depression are and offers treatment options including talk therapy, yoga, and, with a physician's participation, antidepressant medication. The patients are "happy to talk, as long as you stay away from the idea of mental illness," said Dr. Sudipto Chatterjee, a psychiatrist involved in the program.[8]

When we finally abolish the stigma associated with anxiety, the benefit will be twofold: not only will people be more willing to be treated for chronic, pervasive anxiety; they will also be better educated about how managing their anxiety can help them maintain their health. Because that is the proverbial rock-bottom line: managing your anxiety is good for your health. Even if we don't know for sure that anxiety causes disease, we do know that managing anxiety goes a long way toward managing the symptoms of disease. When people are able to acknowledge without embarrassment the role that anxiety plays in their illness, they can learn to understand anxiety well enough to control their symptoms and perhaps even the course of their illness.

NADINE: "THIS DISEASE IS JUST A FACT OF LIFE, AND I JUST KEEP ON MOVING AND IGNORE IT"

Which brings me to Nadine, a sixty-one-year-old dean of undergraduates at a large state university. Married and the mother of two grown children, Nadine has for the last seventeen years been living with fibromyalgia, a chronic pain condition whose symptoms include widespread pain in muscles, ligaments, and tendons; various and multiple tender points—places on the body that, when even gentle pressure is applied, cause pain; sleep disturbances; and fatigue. Known in the past as fibrositis, chronic muscle pain syndrome, psychogenic rheumatism, and tension myalgias, fibromyalgia affects more women than men and has been receiving significant attention in recent years, not only because of how many people it affects—between 3 and 6 percent of Americans, according to the National Fibromyalgia Association (NFA)—but also because of controversy surrounding its legitimacy as a disease.

As NFA President Lynne Matallana asserted at ADAA's 2008 national conference, the condition is very real, despite some dubiousness within the medical community. Matallana, who co-founded the NFA with Karen Lee Richards in 1997 after the women met through an online fibromyalgia chat group, says they started the organization to provide sufferers with information and support they desperately needed. Part of the issue, both then and now, is that there is no specific laboratory test that can be administered to a patient to diagnose the condition. Physicians rely on patients' descriptions of their symptoms to form a fibromyalgia diagnosis, the guidelines for which were first established in 1990 by Frederick Wolfe, M.D., director of the National Databank for Rheumatic Diseases. But a January 2008 story in *The New York Times* quotes Dr. Wolfe as saying he has become "cynical and discouraged about the diagnosis [and] now considers the condition a physical response to stress, depression, and economic and social anxiety."[9] Other physicians are skeptical as well: Nortin M. Hadler, M.D., professor of medicine at the University of North Carolina and also quoted in the *Times,* believes that being diagnosed with fibromyalgia makes people feel worse by encouraging them to think of themselves as sick. "These people live under a cloud," he said. "And the more they seem to be around the medical establishment, the sicker they get."[10] This is not surprising coming from Dr. Hadler, an outspoken critic of what he calls the American health care system's growing tendency to overdiagnose and overtreat as illnesses what he sees as the inevitable aches, pains, and discomforts of life. As with most medical conundrums, there are (at least) two sides, and on the other one is Daniel J. Clauw, M.D., professor of medicine at the University of Michigan, who reports that brain scans of fibromyalgia patients show that they process pain differently than do people without the disorder.[11] As of this writing, several pharmaceutical firms have already received approval from the Food and Drug Administration to market either new or existing medications as treatments for fibromyalgia. And numerous reputable websites, such as that of the Mayo Clinic, feature detailed discussions of symptoms, diagnosis, treatments, coping skills, and other aspects of the condition.

What matters in the context of our discussion is the role that anxiety plays in either triggering or exacerbating fibromyalgia, which brings me back to Nadine. The symptoms started when she was in her mid-forties.

"I developed this backache that wouldn't go away. The pain radiated from the middle of my back all the way down. It was especially bad right around where my bra pressed into my skin. I thought maybe I needed to exercise—I wasn't doing anything at the time—so I started going to the campus recreation center whenever I could. I tried aerobics, stretching, working out on the machines; we even bought a new mattress, but nothing worked. I began to wake up in the middle of the night because it hurt so much where my body touched the mattress. It got so I never slept through the night anymore, and I started walking around like a zombie. This went on for months.

"So I went to the doctor. I was very fortunate to have a young and progressive female physician who was very well informed. She did a lot of tests and asked me a lot of questions and, after ruling out a bunch of other things, said she thought I had fibromyalgia. There was no test for it but if you had constant pain for at least three months, which I did, and at least ten or eleven sensitive spots on your body where if you press even a little it hurts—which I also did—the doctor said you met the diagnostic criteria for the disease."

Nadine says there's no one thing that triggers an episode of particularly bad pain, but she carries her tension mostly in her neck and shoulders (as many of us do), and when she's anxious or stressed, this area tightens and triggers pain in other parts of her body.

"If I'm stressed because I have to meet a deadline or because I've just learned that the state legislature is cutting our budget again, my muscles tense and it inevitably causes my fibromyalgia to flare. And that means I've absolutely got to get out and work my body. And I can't slack off and make it up later: if I don't exercise for a week, I'll get so stiff, I'll barely be able to walk.

"Exercise is crucial to controlling this thing. I have to work out every day, especially if I'm feeling anxious or under pressure. I get on the treadmill every morning because I want to get my endorphins going. My husband and I like being outdoors, but my

back will spasm out if I start walking without warming up first, so when we decide to do some hiking, for example, I have to do a level walk first. It's just an adjustment I've made: if I want to do something strenuous, I warm up first. If I'm traveling, I wake up earlier to fit my exercise in. I don't always feel like doing it; when you're in pain, it's hard to motivate yourself to get on the treadmill. But if I don't, my muscles tighten more and more and then I get a bad attack and it's that much harder to recover.

"I don't like taking medication; the side effects of some of the drugs sound worse than the illness. I exercise a lot because I prefer to do this without depending on pills, especially if I have to take them for the rest of my life. But I know other people with fibromyalgia who think differently than I do. Some of them want pills, and that's fine for them. But my job entails a lot of stress and I have to physically work it out of my body. I'm not always able to leave my work behind at the end of the day; I spend a lot of time in meetings and bring home tons of paperwork, and I sit a lot and work at the computer a lot and my body ends up in knots. So I do my exercise whether I want to or not. This disease is just a fact of life, and I just keep on moving and ignore it."

What I find most striking about Nadine is that she is empowered, not hampered, by acknowledging the role that anxiety plays in her illness. Rather than retreat from her career, she maintains a rigorous exercise schedule to diffuse the effects of working. Rather than quit hiking because she's afraid it might adversely affect her body, she warms up by walking and prepares her body for the exertion to come. Rather than succumb to pain and fatigue by retiring from life, she pushes on into its midst, saying she ignores the illness. The way I see it, what Nadine is ignoring is not the illness but the discomfort of its symptoms; she is mindful of the illness and respectful of the depredations it can wreak upon her body just as a skilled swimmer is mindful and respectful of the ocean: each acknowledges the unconquerable force of what surrounds her and channels her exertions toward going with the flow. Each stays afloat by accepting the physical reality in which

she is suspended and, by deploying strength, intelligence, and discipline, survives and even flourishes. If ever there were someone who illustrated the saying that knowledge is power, Nadine is it.

Thus I can say with confidence that managing your anxiety is good for your health. The rest of this chapter comprises a list of some other illnesses that research is showing to have a significant connection with anxiety.

Cardiovascular disease. As I mentioned earlier, studies have shown that the anxiety and tension of being in a bad marriage make it more likely that a woman will have either a heart attack or other cardiovascular problem. And there's more: it seems that women with phobic anxiety are more likely to die of heart illness than women with fewer or no anxieties. An ongoing study of more than 72,000 female nurses that began in 1976 and is tracking their health over time found that those who had high levels of phobic anxiety were 59 percent more likely to die of heart disease, particularly sudden cardiac death (abrupt, unforeseen loss of heart function), than those who did not have phobic anxiety.[12] But psychology is not destiny: JoAnn Manson, M.D., one of the lead investigators of the Nurses' Health Study, reminds us that correcting poor lifestyle habits can lower the incidence of coronary artery disease in both women and men by a whopping *83 percent.*[13] If that's not enough to get you to quit smoking and start exercising a few days a week, well, it should be.

Asthma. This has become more common over the last twenty years or so and is emerging as having links to a variety of psychological disorders. Anxiety in asthma patients isn't new; the sensation of being unable to get enough air makes everyone anxious, whether she or he has asthma or not. What is new is the idea that an asthma patient's anxiety may not be a direct result of the asthma but a separate problem that coexists with the asthma and exacerbates its symptoms. This idea is supported in part by the results of a 2003 joint study by American and German scientists

that looked at more than four thousand people between the ages of eighteen and sixty-five and found that both participants who were suffering from severe asthma at the time of the study and those who had a history of lifetime severe asthma, although not having an episode at the time of the study, were more likely to suffer from an anxiety disorder.[14] The data hold true for children as well: anxiety and depressive disorders are nearly twice as common in young people with asthma as they are in young people without asthma.[15]

Accelerated breast cancer recurrence. There seems to be a connection between long-term stress and a more rapid recurrence of breast cancer. A 2007 University of Rochester study of ninety-four women whose tumors had recurred found that those with previous histories of trauma or prolonged, intense stress were likely to see their tumors recur more rapidly than women who reported no stressful experiences (aside from living with breast cancer, of course). The women who had histories of trauma (for example, rape, suicide of a family member, life-threatening injury, or childhood sexual abuse) had, on average, a two-and-a-half-year disease-free interval before their tumors recurred; the women who experienced intense stress (resulting from dealing with the death of a parent, divorce, or living through an earthquake, for example) had a disease-free interval of just over three years. But the tumors of women who reported neither trauma nor intense stress typically did not recur until about five years had passed. Oxana Palesh, Ph.D., lead author of the study, said it clearly demonstrated that it is "important to recover from trauma or stressful events for your mental and physical health."[16] For the sake of clarity, I want to emphasize that these findings should not be interpreted to mean that feeling anxious or stressed will cause breast cancer to recur but rather that, among study participants whose breast cancer *did* recur, having a history of trauma or intense, prolonged stress seemed to hasten the recurrence.

Chronic pain conditions. Whereas depression has long been recognized as a common companion to chronic pain, we have only recently begun to study how anxiety fits into the picture. And it's there: primary care patients who come in complaining of conditions such as muscle pain, stomach pain, or headache are also likely to suffer from anxiety. And people who live with chronically painful conditions such as rheumatoid arthritis, migraine headaches, chronic spinal pain, and fibromyalgia (as mentioned earlier) are also very likely to suffer from an anxiety disorder.[17]

Though it isn't surprising to learn that people who live with pain are also prone to anxiety, what is surprising are new data that suggest that anxiety seems to accompany chronic pain as much as depression and, in some cases, even more. This is significant, as fear and anxiety affect the way a person experiences chronic pain, often intensifying its effects. People with anxiety sensitivity (a condition that causes a person to fear the bodily sensations associated with anxiety in the belief they may have harmful consequences) or chronic anxiety disorders are particularly vulnerable, as they may respond to chronic pain with drastically negative misinterpretations of what the pain means. This may make them afraid that the pain will worsen or return and inspire them to become hypervigilant, which in turn makes them reluctant to move their bodies and risk reinjuring themselves. This commonly perpetuates their belief that they are more disabled than they actually are, creating a vicious circle in which they limit their activities, become more and more isolated, and grow increasingly convinced that their anxiety and fear are well founded.[18]

Eating disorders. Anorexia nervosa, whose sufferers starve themselves to achieve and maintain a body weight that is 85 percent or less of what is considered normal for them, and bulimia nervosa, whose sufferers go on eating binges and afterward seek to counteract the effects by inducing vomiting, using laxatives and diuretics, and exercising compulsively, are serious psychiatric illnesses. The origins of these conditions are currently the focus of energetic debate and research, some of which suggests they may be genetically linked and much of which is showing them to be closely tied to anxiety. Scientists around the world have found that among persons suffering from anorexia and/or bulimia, typically two thirds also suffer from an anxiety disorder.[19] In addition, the anxiety seems to predate the eating disorder: in a study of 672 people with either anorexia, bulimia, or a combination of the two, participants said that their anxiety began when they were children, well before they developed either condition.[20]

The implications are great: anorexia has one of the highest mortality rates of all psychiatric disorders.[21] When you consider that one out of every two hundred American women suffers from anorexia, two to three out of every one hundred American women suffer from bulimia, and that, of the roughly eight million Americans who have an eating disorder, seven million of them are women,[22] it becomes clear that if we can get better at recognizing and treating anxiety disorders in children, we may very well be saving lives ten, twenty, and thirty years down the line.

Obesity. Not surprisingly, research shows a correlation between mental disorders and weight. A German study of 2,064 women aged eighteen to twenty-five found that obese women had the highest rate of psychological disorders overall, and, most strikingly, were much more likely to suffer from an anxiety disorder than women of normal weight.[23]

As with eating disorders, there is evidence that anxiety problems in childhood may render girls vulnerable to obesity later in life. A long-term study of 403 females and 417 males living in New York State began assessing the participants in 1983, when they ranged in age from nine to eighteen. The most recent assessment for which data are currently available occurred in 2003, when the participants were twenty-eight to forty years old. At that time, researchers found that the body mass indexes of the women with anxiety disorders were .13 to .18 percent higher than those of the women without anxiety disorders. Interestingly, the men yielded different results: at no point in the study did a boy's or a man's anxiety disorder influence his body mass index.[24] The researchers concluded that treating anxiety and depression in girls and women may be an effective strategy in the battle against obesity. I could not agree more.

Alcohol and drug abuse. Anxiety and mood disorders are closely associated with alcoholism and other substance abuse. In addition, among people with an alcohol or drug abuse problem, 15 percent also have an independent anxiety disorder—that is, an anxiety disorder that is separate from the substance abuse problem and not a result of it—and 20 percent also have an independent mood disorder (depression, for instance).[25]

These statistics raise an interesting question: If these people developed the anxiety disorder independently of their substance abuse problem and not as a result of it, might it be possible that their substance abuse began as an attempt to deal with their anxiety?

Some scientists think so: Jitender Sareen, M.D., who has analyzed data of several American and Canadian studies, found that, with the exception of generalized anxiety disorder, all the anxiety disorders predated the participants' use of amphetamines and hallucinogens. Which is to say that participants who suffered from panic disorder, agoraphobia, specific phobia, or some forms of social phobia developed these disorders *before* they began using illicit drugs. This led Dr. Sareen and his colleagues to suggest that anxiety might increase a person's vulnerability to using drugs and alcohol and emphasize that clinicians and researchers alike need to develop an awareness of the connection between anxiety and substance use.[26]

You don't have to be a researcher to understand the connection: for many people, having a glass of wine or beer or a cocktail is a pleasant, socially acceptable, and perfectly legal way to relax and distance themselves from the stresses of the day. But if you have an anxiety disorder, imbibing even moderate amounts of alcohol or using illicit drugs can worsen the anxiety symptoms and even trigger a panic attack. The irony is obvious: if you're feeling anxious and have a few beers to take the edge off, you may end up intensifying the anxiety, which may then prompt you to drink even more and catalyze the vicious circle effect.

Let me say once more: the point of this chapter is to arm you, not alarm you. The point is to provide you with the knowledge you need to change some of your ways of being and living so you can be healthier and live better and longer. If bickering with your spouse has become your main way of relating to each other, don't fret about the toll it may already have taken on your heart; instead, start today, now, *this very moment* to work toward resolving your differences in a less contentious way. If you are overwhelmed by the burden of caring for someone with Alzheimer's or another chronic illness, relieve some of the stress by looking into respite care. The Family Caregiver Alliance (www.caregiver.org/caregiver/jsp/home.jsp) and the Alzheimer's Association (www.alz.org/index.asp) both offer resources for caretakers who need a break from their responsibilities (for more contact information, see Resources, page 237).

There is help out there. And, of course, there's the help you can provide yourself. For some ways to get started, I invite you to move on to the Ross Prescription.

nine

THE ROSS PRESCRIPTION, PART I

TAKING INVENTORY

This chapter is designed to help you step back from your anxiety and assess it, observe it, and, once you have done that, manage, modify, and, if necessary, ultimately accept it.

First you will assess your anxiety, identifying what makes you anxious, how you tend to respond, and how the anxiety has affected your life. Then you will observe your anxiety by focusing on how you actually experience it. Finally, you will learn some hands-on, in-the-moment techniques to help you diminish as well as tolerate and coexist with it.

Ready? Okay. Let's go.

ASSESS

Take a few minutes to think about some situations or circumstances that are currently causing you anxiety, worry, or stress or have done so recently. For example, you might have been chronically anxious about your kindergartner's safety ever since the day he got on the wrong school bus and didn't disembark with the other children when it arrived at your stop. Or you may be wracked with anxiety at the prospect of telling your sister that she and her three daughters cannot stay with you over Easter weekend. Or you may be frantic about having to stand up and present your unit's sales figures at the weekly departmental meeting. No matter what is causing your anxiety, list as many triggers as you can think of, without censoring or judging yourself. Use additional paper if necessary.

SITUATIONS AND/OR CIRCUMSTANCES THAT MAKE ME ANXIOUS, FEARFUL,OR WORRIED:

____

____

____

____

____

____

Now select from the list those situations or circumstances you'd like to explore and write them each in the left-hand column of the Assessment Chart that follows. Think carefully about how long you have been bothered by the anxiety, how it has affected your life, how your life would change if the anxiety were eliminated, and what relationship you think you have with the anxiety (reflexive-impulsive, pervasive-adaptive, primitive-preventive, imperative-fugitive). Then write down your responses.

After you've completed the chart, set it aside for at least an hour. Then come back to it and add any additional thoughts you may have. It is important to include even things that may seem embarrassing or trivial; sometimes the things that are most difficult or seem too insignificant to write about are the most important.

ASSESSMENT CHART

Anxiety-provoking situation or circumstance	*How long has this bothered you?*	*How has this anxiety affected your life?*	*How would your life change if this anxiety were eliminated?*	*What relationship do you think you have with this particular anxiety?*

OBSERVE

Now you're going to look at the situations and circumstances you noted in the left-hand column and think about—observe—how you reacted (or tend to react) to the anxiety provoked by each one. What was your immediate response? What was your subsequent response, and did it change after you had a moment to reconsider? What did you end up doing (or what are you doing, or what do you plan to do)? How did things turn out? Are you satisfied? If not, what might you have done differently?

As you mull over these questions, consider others as well: Did you react without thinking or pretend nothing was happening? Did you confront the fear or run away from it? Did you do anything to relieve the anxious feelings? Did you let anyone know what you were going through, or did you keep it to yourself? Finally, do any of the relationship categories apply to your anxiety, or does it lie somewhere in between or beyond them? Note your perceptions and complete the Observation Exercise that follows on page 205. I have included two examples to give you an idea of how I suggest you think about this exercise.

EXAMPLE #1: Marcy, a twenty-seven-year-old account executive who dislikes speaking up in front of her colleagues.

SITUATION: My boss asked me to give a brief presentation to the staff explaining the Graham project.

1. **My immediate response:** How can I get out of this? Maybe Steve will do it for me.
2. **My subsequent response:** Not a great idea. I've had others sub for me before, and it will look obvious if I do it again.
3. **What I did (or plan to do):** I agreed to do it because I was afraid I'd lose my job if I didn't.
4. **How did things turn out? Am I satisfied with the results?** Actually, it went fine. My boss said I did a good job and that he wants me to do it again next month for the Harrison project (maybe it didn't go so well after all!).
5. **If not, what might I have done differently?** I'm pretty satisfied. The one thing I might have done differently is not to have overprepared, like I did this time. It made me more nervous but didn't make me do better.

EXAMPLE #2: Johnna, a thirty-four-year-old homemaker who has difficulty asserting herself in family situations.

SITUATION: My sister Deirdre has informed me that she and the kids will be staying with us when they come for Easter, but we don't have room for them.

1. **My immediate response:** Ugh! I can't believe this is happening again! I hinted to Deirdre over the phone that our house was pretty full and she freaked out, said I was making it impossible for her to be with the family for Easter. But Craig already told his brother he can stay in the guest room with Shelly and the baby. I feel horrible and guilty. How can I keep my sister away? Asked Craig if Larry and Shelly can stay in a hotel; now he's mad, says I always favor my family over his and we shouldn't break our promise to his brother. We don't have room for four more people. But how can I do this to my sister?
2. **My subsequent response:** Craig is right: it isn't fair to always put Deirdre ahead of his brother—and everyone else, for that matter. He also says that I'm not keeping Deirdre away; I'm only saying we don't have room for her and the kids to stay at our house. He says it doesn't mean we don't care about her, just that we can't have everyone stay over at the same time. My common sense tells me he's right, but I still feel guilty. Deirdre's really mad and the holiday's getting screwed up and I'm stuck in the middle. For a change.
3. **What I did (or plan to do):** I called Deirdre and told her it would be really crowded with her and the kids in the house and mentioned this new hotel with a great indoor pool just down the road. She said it was cold to tell her to stay in a hotel, and besides she couldn't afford it. I told her we'd help pay, but she said that wasn't the point and hung up on me.
4. **How did things turn out? Am I satisfied with the results?** Don't know yet. Easter is next weekend, and I haven't heard anything. Stomach in knots; Craig losing patience with me. Afraid to call Deirdre; maybe she'll call me? Big mess.
5. **If not, what might I have done differently?** Don't know.

Now get a pen and, using your own experiences, answer the following questions (use additional paper if you need more room):

Observation Exercise

Select an anxiety-provoking situation from the Assessment Chart and write it down.

SITUATION:

Now answer each of the questions that follow. You can answer them in your head, but most people say that writing them down helps them figure out what the thoughts and feelings signify.

1. **My immediate reaction:**

2. **My subsequent reaction:**

3. **What I did (or plan to do):**

4. **How did things turn out? Am I satisfied with the results?**

5. **If not, what might I have done differently?**

ACCEPT

Once you have assessed the nature of your anxiety and looked at how you interact with it, you begin to have options: you can change the way you relate to anxiety-provoking situations, you can take steps to diffuse the anxious feelings, and/or you can learn to tolerate and ultimately accept that worry, anxiety, and stress are an inevitable part of life. To which end I offer an invaluable tool for dealing with the inevitable: the Eight Points: Techniques to Control Anxiety, Worry, and Stress.

I first heard about these gems from the late, great Manuel Zane, M.D., one of the pioneers in treating phobias and panic attacks. He had developed a set of techniques that he called the Six Points to help his patients stay grounded when in the grip of intense anxiety. The Points were simple, concrete directives to help patients focus on what was happening in the moment rather than what their imaginations feared might happen. This enabled them to modify the essence of the experience from fleeing fear to confronting it.

Over time, I took the liberty of adding two points and modifying the others for use with my own patients as well as for people who asked me for help getting their everyday anxiety under control. They remain simple, solid steps that anyone can take anytime, anywhere, to remain grounded when anxiety threatens to throw them off balance.

The Eight Points: Techniques to Control Anxiety, Worry, and Stress

1. Expect, allow, and accept that worry, anxiety, and stress are part of life.
2. When you feel yourself getting anxious or starting to worry, stop, breathe, and think.
3. Focus on what you can do, rather than on what you cannot do.
4. Label your anxiety level from 1 to 10, with 10 being the highest. Note the thoughts and behaviors you have at this level

and what happens to the level when you change your thoughts and behaviors.

5. Ask yourself: "What am I really anxious about?"
6. Ask yourself: "What can I do to lower my anxiety level?"—and do it.
7. Stay rooted in the here and now. Focus on the information you have rather than on the "what if?"s that often accompany anxiety.
8. Expect, allow, and accept that worry, anxiety, and stress will return, because they are part of life.

To help you get a sense of how the Eight Points work, I'll go through them and offer examples of how they might be used.

POINT 1: EXPECT, ALLOW, AND ACCEPT THAT WORRY, ANXIETY, AND STRESS ARE PART OF LIFE. For this one, it's helpful to compose an acceptance statement that verbalizes your acceptance of uncomfortable, anxiety-related feelings, such as:

a. I give myself permission to feel uneasy when I walk into a room full of people I don't know.
b. I can tolerate the anxiety I feel when I walk by my teenager's horrible, messy, smelly, chaotic bedroom.
c. It's okay not to fall asleep the moment my head hits the pillow.
d. It's acceptable to feel stressed out while waiting for the results of my blood test to come in.
e. In Johnna's case: Dealing with my sister is often stressful. I've gotten through it before and I'll get through it again.

POINT 2: WHEN YOU FEEL YOURSELF GETTING ANXIOUS OR STARTING TO WORRY, STOP, BREATHE, AND THINK. When we're feeling anxious, we often react automatically, without thinking. When you become aware that your anxiety level is rising, stop the automatic reaction by taking two or three slow, deep breaths and asking yourself, "What are my instincts telling me to do?" And, "What should I do? What can I do?"

In Johnna's case, her instincts told her to avoid upsetting her sister at any cost. Had she asked herself what she should or could do, she might have instead resisted the temptation to placate Deirdre, which she knew from experience would do no good, and might even backfire (which it did).

POINT 3: FOCUS ON WHAT YOU CAN DO, RATHER THAN ON WHAT YOU CANNOT DO. When people tell me they can't do something, whether it's a phobia patient saying he can't drive over a bridge or a friend saying she can't eat dinner alone in a restaurant, I tell them to take the "t" off the word "can't," implying that they *can* do it—it's just that it may be difficult. For example, when someone says, "I can't drive over a bridge," I suggest that he or she say, "I *can* drive over a bridge, with difficulty." Or instead of "I can't eat dinner alone in a restaurant," I suggest "I *can* eat dinner alone in a restaurant, but it makes me anxious when I do it." Saying "I can" doesn't mean it's easy; it means it's possible. That's the point here: doing what is possible, even if it isn't comfortable.

In Johnna's case, she was focusing on what she could not do: "I can't tell my sister that there's no room for her and her kids"—because she was anticipating Deirdre's anger and trying to avert a conflict. Had I been counseling her, I would have told her to remove the "t" and focus on the *can:* "I *can* tell my sister that there's no room for her and her kids because we've already committed to hosting Larry's family. I *can* also suggest alternate accommodations and offer to help her pay for them. What I cannot do is stop her from being angry." And I would urge her to go one step further and say, "I *can* live with the discomfort of knowing that Deirdre is angry with me."

POINT 4: LABEL YOUR ANXIETY LEVEL FROM 1 TO 10, WITH 10 BEING THE HIGHEST. NOTE THE THOUGHTS AND BEHAVIORS YOU

HAVE AT THIS LEVEL AND WHAT HAPPENS TO THE LEVEL WHEN YOU CHANGE YOUR THOUGHTS AND BEHAVIORS. This one makes you more aware both of the fact that your anxiety moves up and down and that you can interrupt the anxiety spiral by identifying and changing what you think about and what you do.

In Johnna's case, had she labeled her level while in the midst of her phone call with Deirdre, she would probably have put it at a 7 or 8. During that tense conversation, Johnna's thoughts veered toward worst-case scenarios: "I'm a terrible sister"; "Deirdre will be furious with me"; "My sister will never talk to me again." Had she stopped for a moment, taken a deep breath, and challenged these dire predictions by asking herself, "Do I really believe I'm a terrible sister? Do I really think that Deirdre will never speak to me again?," she would have seen her anxiety level start to drop.

POINT 5: ASK YOURSELF: "WHAT AM I REALLY ANXIOUS ABOUT?" For this one, establish whether your anxiety is triggered by a real threat to your well-being or that of a loved one or by the distorted thinking we commonly engage in when we're in a state of emotional arousal. Some types of distorted thinking are:

a. **Catastrophic thoughts:** For instance, "If I mess up on the staff presentation, I'll get fired"; or, in Johnna's case, "If I don't let my sister stay with me, I'll never see her or my nieces again."
b. **Overgeneralizations:** "No one ever, *ever* does *anything* to help around the house!"; or "If I let my kids eat *anything* that isn't organically grown, they're going to have health problems down the road."
c. **All-or-nothing thinking:** "If I don't look absolutely perfect tonight, he won't call me again"; or "If I don't get all the Christmas decorations up on time, it'll ruin the holiday for my family."
d. **Jumping to conclusions:** "My biopsy results aren't back

yet, and it's been a whole day—something must be terribly wrong"; or "My father's over thirty minutes late, and he's usually so prompt—he must have had an accident or a heart attack."

POINT 6: ASK YOURSELF: "WHAT CAN I DO TO LOWER MY ANXIETY LEVEL?"—AND DO IT. Think about Point 5, in which you considered what you were really anxious about. If distorted thinking is causing your anxiety, challenge the assumptions behind the distortions: Might not your biopsy results be delayed because of the long holiday weekend? Is there any evidence that your family's Christmas will go to rack and ruin if some of the decorations go up late? (Most likely no one will notice.) Debunking faulty assumptions is often the first step toward dissipating anxiety. And whether the anxiety is precipitated by distorted thinking or by realistic fears and concerns—say, your teenager, who just got his license, is out with the car at night for the first time—the anxiety-lowering techniques in Chapter 10 will help calm you down. Once you develop a supply of anxiety-lowering techniques, learn to trust them, even if in the midst of a stressful episode you don't think anything will work. For example, if a certain breathing or relaxation exercise has worked for you in the past but you feel so anxious that you can't imagine ever calming down, try doing it anyway.

POINT 7: STAY ROOTED IN THE HERE AND NOW. FOCUS ON THE INFORMATION YOU HAVE RATHER THAN THE "WHAT IF?"S THAT OFTEN ACCOMPANY ANXIETY. When you find yourself playing out worst-case scenarios in your mind, as in "What if my company doesn't get the new account because I couldn't close the deal?" or "What if the doctor tells me the mole on my back is malignant?" or "What if I forget my boss's name when I introduce her to my fiancé tomorrow night?," ask yourself: "What valid information do I currently have about the situation?" and respond to that, rather than try to predict the future (which many of us do when we feel uncertain about something we're concerned about). For example, tell yourself: "Even if I can't close the deal, it will still be on the table" or "The dermatologist assured me that 80 percent of the moles he removes are benign" or "My boss is always forgetting people's names and joking about it—if anyone will be sympathetic, she will."

POINT 8: EXPECT, ALLOW, AND ACCEPT THAT WORRY, ANXIETY, AND STRESS WILL RETURN, BECAUSE THEY ARE PART OF LIFE. We have come full circle (see Point 1).

ten

THE ROSS PRESCRIPTION, PART 2

TAKING ACTION

This chapter offers concrete actions—exercises, techniques, and suggestions for what to do—for combating unwanted responses to anxiety. Some require pen and paper (or keyboard and screen); others, willpower and a vivid imagination. All of them are worth stowing in your antianxiety arsenal.

WHAT TO DO . . . WHEN YOU WANT TO AVOID OR FLEE SOMEONE OR SOMETHING BUT KNOW YOU SHOULD STAY AND TOUGH IT OUT

Remember Stan, the guy whose catastrophic thinking led him from picturing himself having a panic attack to picturing himself being incarcerated in a mental hospital? And Holly, the young woman who worked as a barista to avoid interviewing for a graphic designer position? This exercise worked for them, and it may very well work for you, too.

Exercise 1

Think of an anxiety-provoking situation that made you want to avoid or flee it, then fill in the blanks:

The worst thing that could happen if I were to confront or remain in this situation is ____________.

And then ____________;

And then ____________;

And then ____________;

And then ____________;

And then ____________;

And then ____________;

And then ____________;

And then ____________;

And then ____________;

And then ____________.

When you have reached the final "and then," consider the probability of it actually happening. Chances are it will be very remote indeed.

Exercise 2

This exercise asks you to reverse the process you followed in the last one: rather than ride the anxiety rocket to a preposterous extreme, you're going to dismantle it into components so it can't go anywhere. Using the space provided or additional paper if you need it, answer the following questions:

1. Describe a time when you either avoided or fled a situation because you overestimated its potential for discomfort or awkwardness.

   ____

   ____.

2. What thoughts contributed to your avoiding or fleeing the situation?

   ____

   ____.

3. What was the worst thing you thought might happen if you confronted the situation?

   ____

   ____.

4. What evidence do you have that this worst thing could happen? For example, has it happened in the past?

   ____

   ____.

5. Considering your answer to Question 4, what do you now believe was the worst thing that might have happened had you confronted the situation?

   ____

   ____.

6. Imagine this situation arising again. Do you picture yourself handling it differently next time? If your answer is yes, what would you do? If no, why not?

   ____

   ____.

WHAT TO DO . . . WHEN YOUR BODY IS ANXIOUS AND YOU WANT TO CALM IT DOWN

As you know, anxiety can make your body behave in unexpected and inconvenient ways. Here are some things you can do to calm your pounding heart, unknot your muscles, and ease some of those disconcerting physiological symptoms without anyone being the wiser.

PHYSIOLOGICAL REACTION	SOME WAYS TO HANDLE IT
Pounding heart	Give the pounding a rhythm. Think of a song with a heavy bass line, and imagine singing or playing along with it. Have fun with it. Try squeezing your toes or tapping your foot along with the beat.
Lightheadedness	Pay attention to your breathing, making sure your breaths are neither too deep nor too shallow, and that you're not holding your breath. Practice the diaphragmatic breathing technique described in the section following this chart.
Hot flushes, cold sweats, copious perspiration	Imagine holding ice cubes in your hands. Picture the toxins flowing out of your body. Take a drink of cold water. If your face feels hot and flushed, imagine it's just your natural youthful, rosy glow (with no danger of sun damage).
Trembling, shaky hands	Rather than try to stop your hands from shaking, give them permission to do the opposite: let them shake even more. Try shaking them continuously for three minutes without stopping (I bet you can't do it). Notice how the shaking dissipates when you eliminate the stress of trying to prevent it.

PHYSIOLOGICAL REACTION	SOME WAYS TO HANDLE IT
Butterflies in stomach	Give them shapes, sizes, and colors. Imagine them flying in formation. Make them dance with one another. Play with the colors, patterns, and movement.
Muscle tension	Start with your feet and work your way up the body, clenching and releasing each muscle group as you go. Clench your toes in your shoes, your hands in your pockets, and the rest as you can. No one can see you do this and it really does help.

WHAT TO DO . . . WHEN YOU WANT TO QUIET YOUR NERVES AND SIMPLY RELAX

Relaxation Technique: Breathe Away Tension

Breathing slowly and deeply from the diaphragm is a highly effective tool for reducing tension, stress, and the body-knotting, heart-pumping effects of anxiety. Most of us don't give much thought to how we breathe. Yet our breathing habits—particularly when we are feeling stressed, anxious, or frightened—can profoundly affect the way we feel, by either increasing the tension we feel or diminishing it. For example, if you tend to hold your breath when you feel stressed, the muscles in your body may tense and tighten, making you feel stiff and even lightheaded. Or, if you overbreathe when you're anxious, you may feel as if you're beginning to hyperventilate, thereby increasing your anxiety. Breathing diaphragmatically with long, smooth, deep breaths will encourage you to release your muscles, enable the exchange of oxygen and carbon dioxide to happen naturally and in the proper proportions, and make you feel more calm and relaxed.

While you may have to concentrate on the mechanics of diaphragmatic breathing at first, after a while you may find yourself using it automatically when you are faced with a stressful situation.

In addition to learning to breathe from your diaphragm, you may find it helpful to become aware of your natural breathing styles when you are relaxed and when you are feeling anxious. To help you think this through, complete the following sentences:

When I am relaxed, my breathing is (check all that apply):

❑ slow ❑ rapid ❑ normal

❑ deep ❑ shallow ❑ relaxed

❑ from the stomach ❑ from the chest ❑ from the diaphragm

When I feel anxious or stressed, my breathing is most likely to be (check all that apply):

❑ slow ❑ rapid ❑ normal

❑ deep ❑ shallow ❑ relaxed

❑ from the stomach ❑ from the chest ❑ from the diaphragm

When I feel anxious or stressed, I am most likely to (check one):

❑ hold my breath ❑ overbreathe ❑ sigh repeatedly

Familiarize yourself with your breathing patterns and notice what happens to your anxiety levels when you alter the way you breathe. If you typically breathe quickly, try slowing down your breathing the next time you feel anxious; if you tend to take small, shallow breaths, try breathing more deeply, expanding your abdomen outward as you inhale.

Experiment with what works for you. Many of my panic disorder patients report that they can lessen the intensity of a panic attack or even avert one altogether by focusing on breathing diaphragmatically. If it works for them, it can work for you.

How to Breathe Diaphragmatically

- Begin by loosening your clothes and lying down.
- Once you are lying down, find a comfortable and relaxed position and take a few seconds to slow your breathing.
- When your breathing has slowed, inhale through your nose, expanding your belly and filling it with air as if it were a balloon. Then collapse your belly, exhaling through your mouth. As you do this, keep your chest as still as you can.
- Place a book on your belly and practice making it go up and down with your breathing. It should go up on the inhale and down on the exhale. This may seem counterintuitive at first, but keep at it.
- After you have been practicing for a while, remove the book and continue breathing the same way. Put your left hand on your upper chest and your right hand on your belly. Your left hand should be still, and your right hand should move up and down.
- As you inhale, practice expanding your abdomen like a balloon. As you exhale, slowly release your abdomen and let your diaphragm push the air out of your lungs.
- Continue to breathe slowly and smoothly, prolonging your exhale even more than your inhale.
- Remember: When you inhale, breathe in through your nose, and when you exhale, breathe out through your mouth. Emphasize the exhalation by making a long hissing sound—"ssssssssssss"—leaving your mouth open and relaxed.

WHAT TO DO . . . WHEN YOU GET INTO AN ARGUMENT WITH YOUR HUSBAND, BOYFRIEND, OR PARTNER, AND YOU WANT TO PROTECT YOUR HEALTH

If you're the type of woman who squelches her feelings during a fight, you're not doing yourself any favors: as you may recall, the Framingham Study found that women who kept their feelings to themselves during marital disagreements were four times as likely to die within a ten-year follow-up period as women who spoke their minds.[1] Thus I strongly recommend:

- **When you and your spouse are fighting, express yourself.** Tell him what's going on inside you. Get it out there. Be honest and authentic and genuine, even if it isn't easy. It's no secret that women are often reluctant to voice their feelings for fear of alienating or wounding their partners: What if he gets angry? What if he walks out? What if I hurt his feelings? But to them I say: It's better to risk losing his affection for a few hours or even days, or to tolerate your discomfort at seeing him sulk, than to risk compromising your health over the long haul. That said, when you do express yourself, be civil: you have nothing to gain by slinging verbal razor blades and slashing his feelings to ribbons. One way to maintain civility is to express yourself in terms of what you feel rather than blaming or accusing him. For example, it's more effective to say "I was really hurt tonight when you made fun of my haircut in front of my colleagues" than to sally forth with "How dare you humiliate me in front of the people I work with? You were a real creep tonight!" Accusing him in this way is likely to make him feel attacked and obliged to launch a counteroffensive, whereas if you restrict your comments to how *you* feel, he has less need to defend himself. Finally, the temporary anxiety you may experience about telling your spouse what you're really feeling is small stuff compared to the long-term benefits your heart and health will gain.

PHYSICAL AND MENTAL TECHNIQUES, ACTIVITIES, AND EXERCISES TO EASE ANXIETY AND TENSION AND HELP YOU RELAX

1. **Sit in a chair and let your body go limp.** Let your arms hang, release your stomach muscles, allow your head to drop forward toward your chest. Rotate your head clockwise, slowly and gently, until your right ear is over your right shoulder; continue in the same direction until your head is tilted back, then continue until your left ear is over your left shoulder, then continue until your head is dropped forward, as you started. Repeat going in the opposite direction as you begin to . . .
2. **Focus on your breathing.** Breathing from your diaphragm, picture a ball moving up and down inside your abdomen as you inhale and exhale, slowly and evenly. Give the ball color and texture; mentally increase and decrease its size. Play with the image, making the ball spin swiftly, slowly, or not at all.
3. **Picture a place where you would love to be**—it might be a cabin in the mountains, a beach on Kauai, or your grandmother's apartment in Chicago—just pick a place that, when you think about it, makes you feel good. Then imagine yourself in that place, experiencing it, using all your senses to create your surroundings: What colors do you see? What sounds do you hear? What do you smell, feel, taste?
4. **Repeat an encouraging phrase to yourself, over and over again, like a mantra.** For instance, tell yourself: "I've had these anxious thoughts (or feelings) before and they've passed. They'll pass again" or "That which doesn't kill me makes me stronger" (one of my favorites). Some people refer to these kinds of statements as affirmations; others, as positive self-talk. Whatever you call them, they are good for calming yourself down and reminding yourself that you are not powerless, even though you may feel that way at that moment.
5. **If you feel overwhelmed, ask yourself: "Who am I really doing this for?"** If you're volunteering at school, chairing the

prom committee, and coaching the swim team, ask yourself: "Am I doing this for my child? Am I enjoying it?" If the answer is yes, then continue what you're doing. But if you're doing all these things to prove to others (or to yourself) what a hands-on, attentive mother you are, you might do well to drop a few commitments.

6. **Keep a stress management diary.** Keep a small pad handy and make a note of when you feel anxious or stressed (you may want to use some of the categories from the personal habits diary on pages 96–97). Jot down the time of day, where you are, what you're doing. Note where and how the anxiety manifests itself: Is it in your stomach? Your neck? Your head? Your temper? Look for patterns in the entries. When you get a sense of when and why your anxiety or stress gets started, ask yourself what you might be able to do to avert or ease it. Look for things that you enjoy doing and that are realistic options. And give yourself permission to take time to do whatever you need to do to feel better. Women tend to feel guilty about doing things for themselves, but if we make time to build stress-relieving activities into our lives, not only do we feel better, we are more effective both at home and at work. Don't just talk about it—*do it.* Schedule it into your day like any other commitment.
7. **Do something that takes your mind away from thoughts of what you do all the time.** Take up a musical instrument (when I need to destress, I sit down at the piano). Join a chorus or sign up for dance lessons; work in the garden; lose yourself in a jigsaw, crossword, or Sudoku puzzle; cook a new dish you've been wanting to try; knit, crochet, or cross-stitch; take up archery; sign up for a beading workshop or a foreign language class. You're still using your mind, only in a different way than you usually do.
8. **Get a massage.** Though a full-body massage by a licensed professional can set you back more than $75 for an hour, there are less costly ways to get one. Some of the larger air-

ports have kiosks offering five- and ten-minute informal neck massages for tensed-up travelers, and a shopping mall near my house has a storefront emporium where you can get a fifteen-minute neck, back, or foot massage for $15, thirty minutes for $30, and so on. You keep your clothes on and there isn't much privacy, but that's all part of the charm. And you can always get a free massage if you can persuade a friend to do it for you (offering to do it for him or her in return is a powerful inducement). There are books and videos available that teach therapeutic massage techniques.

9. **Stretch.** If you can take a stretching class, great. If you can't, stretch your muscles at home, especially after exercising or sitting still for a long time.
10. **Meditate, take a yoga class, or begin a meditative practice at home.** Remember Teresa, who said she was way too stressed to do yoga? If you think you're too stressed to do a meditative-type activity that requires you to sit still, chances are that's *precisely* what you need to do. Meditation helps dissipate anxiety by focusing your attention on thoughts and images other than those that are worrying you. And yoga combines awareness of breathing with strengthening the body through sustaining a series of postures, or asanas. You don't have to be supple to practice yoga, although if you stick with it, you're likely to end up that way. Look into a beginner's class, or, if there isn't one in your area, try learning from a video, audio, or book and practicing at home.

THE ULTIMATE ANXIETY BUSTER: EXERCISE

I'm giving exercise its own heading because I cannot emphasize enough the tremendous benefits you get from doing it. It's not just that exercise makes you stronger, leaner, and fitter and helps prevent high blood pressure, diabetes, and other diseases; a growing body of research is showing that exercise can also reduce anxiety, especially if you're over thirty-five and aren't afraid to push yourself a little. Researchers at the University of Missouri found that women who exercise at high intensity levels enjoy a greater reduction in anxiety symptoms than women who exercise less intensely or not at all—and that these calming effects were twice as potent for thirty-five- to forty-five-year-olds as they were for eighteen- to twenty-year-olds.[2] There's also the story a Ross Center psychiatrist told me of a fifty-year-old woman who came in with social anxiety. A divorced working mother, she had tried cognitive-behavioral therapy and a variety of medications with little success. Then, in an attempt to try something completely different, she joined a marathon-training group and began to run. Not only did she complete a marathon, her anxiety has dissipated to the point that it is no longer an impediment—that is, as long as she keeps running: by maintaining a rigorous training regimen, she is able to manage her anxiety symptoms.

This is not an isolated case: numerous studies suggest that vigorous physical activity may be a low-cost alternative to psychotherapy and medication for people who either cannot afford to get professional help for their anxiety or are reluctant to seek it.[3] And though doctors have known for some time that intense aerobic exercise can quell anxiety symptoms almost as well as medication does, evidence is emerging that a thirty-minute moderate workout can also do the trick. Andreas Ströhle, M.D., a psychiatrist at Charité-University Medicine Berlin, did an experiment in which he divided fifteen volunteers into two groups and had the first walk on treadmills at a moderate rate for thirty minutes and the second spend the time resting quietly in bed. Afterward, each received an injection of a chemical commonly known to trigger panic attacks. The results were unambiguous: the group that had rested had twice the rate of panic attacks as the group that had exercised.[4] If we extrapolate from there—and I believe we can—it's clear that even moderate exercise is effective at alleviating some anxiety symptoms.

Where do you go from here? To the gym, or the running track, or out your front door. Just put on some comfortable shoes with good support and start walking. My internist says that to stay healthy, women ideally should do a total of two hundred minutes of brisk, cardiovascular-stimulating exercise every week; if they can't manage that, a minimum of four thirty-minute sessions a week is also beneficial.

If even that feels overwhelming, here are some tips adapted from the Mayo Clinic's website[5] on how to motivate yourself to exercise when you're feeling too anxious or depressed to do much of anything:

- Enlist the support of your family, friends, and health provider.
- Identify what you enjoy doing.
- Set reasonable goals.
- Address your barriers.
- Prepare for setbacks and obstacles.

eleven

THE ROSS PRESCRIPTION, PART 3

TAKING CHARGE

This chapter provides information that may be helpful should you wish to explore your anxiety beyond the pages of this book. I have included a list of "I" Statements, which I think of as a self-advocacy tool kit; a guide to what therapists' degrees mean; some questions to ask a prospective therapist; and a few words about medications.

"I" STATEMENTS

We would all do well to remind ourselves of these basic unalienable rights, which, when we truly believe they are our rights, will free us from some of our anxieties. As you read through the list, note which ones seem most germane to you, and, if it strikes you as helpful, write them down on sticky notes and post them where they're likely to cross your line of vision and sink into your consciousness.

"I" Statements—Your Rights

- I have the right to make a mistake and be responsible for it.
- I have the right to say no without feeling guilty.
- I have the right to do what will make me happy, as long as it doesn't infringe on the rights of someone else.
- I have the right to ask for help.
- I have the right to feel angry.
- I have the right to feel confused.
- I have the right to ask questions.
- I have the right to not care.
- I have the right to offer no excuses for my behavior.
- I have the right to have my needs respected.
- I have the right to not know the answer.
- I have the right to disagree.
- I have the right to be weak.
- I have the right to cry.
- I have the right to be scared.
- I have the right to not like everybody.
- I have the right to get what I pay for.
- I have the right to ask for what I want, knowing that I may be refused.
- I have the right to be taken seriously.
- I have the right to set my own priorities.
- I have the right to change my mind.
- I have the right to privacy.
- I have the right to seek professional help.
- I have the right to walk away.
- I have the right to assert myself.
- I have the right to *not* assert myself.

FINDING A RIGHT THERAPIST

I say *a* right therapist rather than *the* right therapist because, for any given person, there are any number of competent, qualified, and compatible mental health professionals from whom to choose. That said, it is important that you feel comfortable with any therapist or physician you work with. Finding the right treatment and personal chemistry may involve meeting with more than one candidate. To help you find your way through the maze of providers, here is a list of different kinds of mental health practitioners and what their degrees mean, followed by some questions you may want to ask as you make your decision.

WHAT MENTAL HEALTH PROFESSIONALS' DEGREES MEAN

M.D. (Doctor of Medicine): Psychiatrist. Psychiatrists are physicians who have completed medical school, followed by a four-year clinical residency in psychiatry. Psychiatrists are trained in the biology, medical aspects, diagnostic assessment, and treatment of psychological disorders. In most states (but not all), psychiatrists are the only mental health professionals who can prescribe medication.

Ph.D. (Doctor of Philosophy): Psychologist. Therapists with a Ph.D. degree have completed four to six years of graduate study, which include training in research methods and psychotherapy. Psychologists are trained in diagnostic assessment and treatment of psychological disorders. In addition, they may do psychological testing.

Psy.D. (Doctor of Psychology): Psychologist. Therapists with a Psy.D. degree have also completed four to six years of graduate study focused on training to work in a clinical setting. They are trained in diagnostic assessment and treatment of psychological disorders. Their training is more focused on psychotherapy than on research. They may do psychological testing.

M.A. (Master of Arts) or **M.S. (Master of Science) in Psychology.** Therapists with either an M.A. or M.S. degree in psychology have completed a two- to three-year graduate program with an emphasis on clinical experience and psychotherapy. They are trained in the assessment, diagnosis, and treatment of psychological disorders.

M.S.W. (Master of Social Work): Social Worker. Therapists with an M.S.W. degree have completed a two- to three-year graduate program focused on social work theory, knowledge, methods, and ethics. Social workers are trained to consider their clients in social, economic, and cultural contexts as they perform diagnostic assessments and treat psychological disorders.

Ed.D. (Doctor of Education). Therapists with an Ed.D. degree have completed a four- to six-year graduate program specializing in child development and education. Their primary focus as clinicians is on identifying and treating developmental problems, as well as educational assessment and planning.

The following initials refer to licensure by state professional boards. They usually follow initials that indicate an academic degree in psychology, social work, or education, as in "Jerilyn Ross, M.A., LICSW."

LCSW	Licensed Clinical Social Worker
LISW	Licensed Independent Social Worker
LICSW	Licensed Independent Clinical Social Worker
CSW–C	Certified Social Worker–Clinical
MFT	Marriage and Family Therapist
MFCC	Marriage, Family, and Child Counselor

Questions to Ask a Prospective Therapist

- What experience and training do you have in treating anxiety and anxiety disorders?

- What is your basic approach to treatment?
- Can you prescribe and monitor medication or refer me to someone who can if that proves necessary?
- How long is the course of treatment?
- How frequent are treatment sessions, and how long do they last?
- Do you include family members in therapy?
- What is your fee schedule, and do you have a sliding scale for varying financial circumstances?
- Are you qualified for reimbursement by my insurance plan?

MEDICATION

There are numerous ways to deal with anxiety without using medication. That said, many of the forty million Americans with anxiety disorders find medication helpful either on its own or as part of a treatment plan. If you are considering using medication, the best way to begin is with an open and honest discussion with your physician, followed by ongoing evaluation and monitoring.

With so many new medications coming to market and so much new research into how they affect the body, it is critical that you choose a physician who is familiar with the latest developments in the field. Not all doctors are well informed about the kinds of medications and combinations of medications prescribed to treat anxiety. For this reason, I urge you to be direct with your physician and ask whether he or she has had experience prescribing and monitoring the use of these kinds of medications. If the answer isn't a resounding yes, or if your doctor does not have sufficient time to answer your questions, you may need to ask for a referral to another doctor—most likely a psychiatrist—who can prescribe a medication regimen for you and monitor your progress. If you think you need a referral, don't be afraid to ask for one. Though many primary care doctors are knowledgeable and comfortable prescribing psychiatric medications, others would prefer to refer you to someone who has more specialized training and experience in this area.

Tips for Talking with Your Doctor About Medication

- Inform your doctor of all medications you are currently taking, including prescription drugs, over-the-counter formulas, herbal supplements, dietary supplements, and vitamins.
- When your physician prescribes a new medication, make sure you get all the information you need about it. Here are some questions you might want to ask:
    - How will this medication help me?
    - How long does it typically take for the medication to start working?
    - What should I expect when it does start working?
    - What side effects might I experience?
    - If I do have side effects, what should I do? (I suggest you ask for the prescribing physician's after-hours phone number and, if you experience symptoms that concern you, call him or her.)
    - Are there any foods or beverages I should avoid while I'm taking the medication?
    - Is it possible that the new medication will interact with other medications I'm already taking or may take in the future?
    - How often should I take it?
    - When should I take it? (Some medications work best if they are taken in the morning; others have side effects that are minimized if they are taken at bedtime.)
    - Should I take it on an empty stomach or with food?
- Your pharmacist is a good source of information about medications and over-the-counter products and is qualified to advise you about how to take the medication, possible drug interactions, and side effects.

Once you've begun a course of medication, be sure to contact your doctor if you have any new or unusual symptoms, even if you are not sure the medication caused them. And, most important, do not stop taking a medication or change the dosage without consulting the prescribing physician. People sometimes make the mistake of stopping their medication because they're feeling better, not realizing that they're feeling better *because* they're taking the medication. If you stop taking your medication abruptly, not only may some of the anxiety symptoms return, but you may also experience serious withdrawal effects. It is crucial to work closely with your physician and be sure that he or she supervises any changes you make in your medication regimen.

You now have insight into how your different relationships with anxiety affect you; you have considered what changes you might want to make to ease your anxiety; and you are armed with an arsenal of tools and techniques to make those changes.

Remember: There is no right or wrong when it comes to how you relate to your anxiety; there is only the question of whether or not it is working for you. If it's working, fine—keep it. If it isn't working, you know what you have to do.

ACKNOWLEDGMENTS

First and foremost, I want to thank the Ross Center for Anxiety & Related Disorders patients and the friends, family members, and acquaintances whose stories inspired and formed the foundation of this book. I am grateful to these women for their candor and for trusting me with their stories.

I also want to thank the professional staff of the Ross Center, whose specialized clinical skills and commitment to excellence ensure that every patient who walks in the door will receive the best possible care. I am especially grateful to Beth Salcedo, M.D., medical director, and Julie Lewis, Ph.D., who, with the consent of their patients, shared their observations and insights with me, and to Kathy Hogen-Bruen, Ph.D., and Daniel S. Pine, M.D., for taking time to read and offer constructive criticism of various sections of this book. In addition, I owe a debt of gratitude to R. Bruce Lydiard, M.D., Ph.D., for alerting us to (and helping us understand) cutting-edge biological research, and to Gordon M. Cantor, M.D., and William E. Cooke, Ph.D., for their insights into complex scientific concepts.

The past year has held many magical moments of conversation with friends, colleagues, and family members, both mine and my co-writer's, about anxiety and worry. Some occurred during formal interviews, others during serendipitous encounters; but most, if not all, yielded anecdotes, perceptions, and suggestions that found their way into the manuscript. I am grateful to Karen Akers, Hilary Brown, June M. Cantor, Sylvia C. Cantor, Barbara Cohen, Merle Green, Jan Ross, Sharryn Ross, Kendra Sagoff, Sue-Ann Siegel, and Ann Wasserman for sharing gems of insight and wisdom.

My co-writer, Robin Cantor-Cooke, was a joy to work with in every way. Her personal grace, warmth, and sense of humor, along with her remarkable gift for translating complex issues into clear, concise language, were reflected in all aspects of our collaboration. With one keen eye focused on perfection and the other on keeping us moving forward, Robin simply and generously did whatever it took to make this book the best it could be. I am profoundly grateful for the opportunity to collaborate with, learn from, and call my friend someone whom I respect and admire so deeply.

Gail Ross, my literary agent, was a driving force not only in finding the ideal home for this book, but also in helping develop some of its core concepts. She is that rarest of representatives: someone who enjoys the respect and affection of clients and editors alike. I thank and treasure Gail for her professional expertise, intellectual vigor, personal warmth, and irreverent sense of humor. Not only is she a great agent, she's great company.

An author is only as good as her publishing team, and I am fortunate to be working with the best. Libby McGuire, publisher of Ballantine Books, had the vision for a new work about women and anxiety and the graciousness to ask me to write it. Marnie Cochran, editor par excellence, leapt into the project when its original champion, Julia Cheiffetz, left to pursue an irresistible opportunity. Marnie is the editor every writer dreams of: intelligent and highly skilled, she helped shape the manuscript with both a panoramic lens and a microscopic eye for detail. It is immeasurably better for her expertise. Lynn Anderson, our copy editor, deployed her formidable erudition and red pencil to query every rogue comma, colon, and quotation mark, while Beth Pearson supervised the transformation of a stack of marked-up manuscript pages to the clean and polished pages you hold in your hands. I am also indebted to production manager Erin Bekowies, to proofreaders Graham Maby and Melissa Pierson, and to Christina Duffy and Lea Beresford, who provided administrative support. Finally, thanks to Casey Hampton for creating the book's elegant interior design, and to Rebecca Lown for designing a cover that is both cheerful and soothing.

No amount of praise could adequately thank Katie Gilbert, my personal assistant and Ross Center office manager. It would not be possible for me to do everything I do—including writing this book—without Katie's impeccable work ethic and unflagging oversight of all aspects of the practice. I am also grateful to all of the Ross Center's administrative staff, and I offer special thanks to Debra Ramnath and our summer intern, Claire Connolly, for helping with the organizational details of the book.

I am enormously grateful to my colleagues at the Anxiety Disorders Association of America: Alies Muskin, chief operating officer; Jean Kaplan Teichroew, director of communications and public relations; and the entire staff, whose energy, compassion, and dedication make ADAA a beacon of help and hope for millions of people across America and around the world.

A special thank-you goes to Margaret Thomas, who managed the household so Robin and I could work without distraction, and to the staff of Chicken Out Rotisserie, whose succulent roasted chicken legs, savory cranberry relish, and mammoth sweet potatoes motivated us to finish the morning's work so we could take a lunch break.

My father, Raymond Ross, died shortly before I finished writing this book. Oftentimes during the last year, when I was feeling overwhelmed with all the things going on in my life, I would visit him and allow his grateful-to-see-me-smile and wonderful sense of humor to lift me up. I miss him dearly. The love he and my mother, who died three years earlier, shared inspires me every single day.

Growing up with loving parents was the catalyst for the extraordinarily close relationship I share with my brother, Richard, whom I love, respect, and admire as much for our differences as for our similarities (he didn't get the worry gene). His loyalty over the years has been a great comfort to me, as is seeing him so happy with his new bride, Sally Carlson.

Although they were not directly involved in the writing of this book, I must acknowledge the young people who bring so much joy to my life: my niece and nephew, Andrea and Justin Ross, who continue to swell my heart with pride; my grandchildren, Chase, Ryan, and Dayna Siegel, and Daniele, Amanda, Morgan, and Derrick Cohen, whose hugs and smiles make my world shine (with special thanks to their parents, Sue-Ann and Eric, Alan and Patricia, and Craig and Kim, for so warmly welcoming me into their lives fourteen years ago); and to Robin's children, Harrison and Graham, who graciously allowed me to hijack their mom for days at a time.

Finally: I could not have written this book without the unwavering encouragement and support of my husband, Ron Cohen, whose intelligence, acumen, grit, and integrity are surpassed only by his generous heart. Thank you, Ronnie, for being my rock: the love of my life, my best friend, and the steadfast knight of my impossible dream.

RESOURCES

ANXIETY DISORDERS ASSOCIATION OF AMERICA

Since 1980, tens of thousands of people suffering with anxiety problems—as well as their family members—have benefited from the services, programs, and publications of the Anxiety Disorders Association of America (ADAA).

ADAA is the leading nonprofit organization solely dedicated to promoting the prevention, early recognition, and treatment of anxiety and related disorders. The volunteer and professional staff of ADAA is devoted to improving the lives of all who suffer from anxiety-related conditions by disseminating information, supporting and promoting research, linking those who need treatment with those who provide it, and educating health professionals, legislators, the media, and the public that *anxiety and related disorders are real, serious, and treatable.*

The association offers programs and resources for physicians and other mental health therapists, individuals who are coping with an anxiety disorder and their family members, and others who are interested in learning about the field.

As one of the founders of the organization, I am very proud of all that ADAA has accomplished in the nearly thirty years of its existence and want to encourage you to take advantage of its many excellent publications and programs.

To learn more about the ADAA, go to www.adaa.org. For general inquiries, send an email to information@adaa.org or call 240-485-1001. ADAA is located at 8730 Georgia Avenue, Suite 600, Silver Spring, MD 20910.

THE ROSS CENTER AND OTHER RESOURCES

If after reading this book and practicing the suggested techniques you are still having difficulty getting your anxiety under control and want to seek therapy, you have many options. Anxiety and related disorders are treated by a wide variety of health professionals, including psychiatrists, psychologists, clinical social workers, and psychiatric nurses. To find a suitable therapist, you may have to meet with more than one to determine whether the two of you are compatible. It is important that you feel comfortable with the therapist you choose to work with.

The life stories you have read about in this book reflect the variety of experiences we find in patients treated at the Ross Center for Anxiety & Related Disorders in Washington, D.C. To learn more about the Ross Center, visit our website at www.rosscenter.com, or call 202-363-1010.

You can obtain a list of additional treatment programs and individual therapists throughout the United States and Canada by contacting the ADAA (for contact information, see page 240).

One way to receive a thorough diagnostic evaluation and treatment for an anxiety or related disorder is to volunteer to participate in a research program. These are often conducted at departments of psychology or psychiatry at universities, medical schools, hospitals, and private mental health facilities. Among these programs are clinical trials whose purpose is to test whether a certain new or experimental treatment—psychological or pharmacological—works for patients with a specific disorder. A major benefit of these studies is that eligible participants receive a free comprehensive evaluation and free or low-cost treatment. These trials usually study a particular type of problem or treatment and may exclude persons with significant medical problems or coexisting psychiatric problems, women of childbearing potential, and persons outside a specified age range.

The National Institutes of Health provides an online registry of federally and privately supported clinical trials in the United States and around the world. For more information, go to www.clinicaltrials.gov.

The following professional and consumer organizations are good resources for information about anxiety and related disorders. I've included organizations representing conditions discussed in the book, as well as others that may be of help and interest to you or your loved ones.

The Alexander Foundation for Women's Health
1700 Shattuck Avenue, Suite 329
Berkeley, CA 94709
510-527-3010
www.afwh.org
contact@afwh.org

Alzheimer's Association
National Office
225 N. Michigan Avenue, 17th Floor
Chicago, IL 60601-7633
312-335-8700
www.alz.org/index.asp
24/7 Helpline for information, referral, and support: 800-272-3900
info@alz.org

American Foundation for Suicide Prevention
120 Wall Street, 22nd Floor
New York, NY 10005
212-363-3500
888-333-AFSP (2377)
www.afsp.org
inquiry@afsp.org

American Medical Women's Association
100 North 20th Street, 4th Floor
Philadelphia, PA 19103
215-320-3716
866-564-2483
www.amwa-doc.org

American Psychiatric Association
1000 Wilson Boulevard, Suite 1825
Arlington, VA 22209-3901
703-907-7300
www.psych.org
apa@psych.org

American Psychological Association
750 First Street, N.E.
Washington, DC 20002-4242
202-336-5500
800-374-2721
www.apa.org

Anxiety Disorders Association of America
8730 Georgia Avenue, Suite 600
Silver Spring, MD 20910
240-485-1001
www.adaa.org
information@adaa.org

Association for Behavioral and Cognitive Therapies (ABCT)
305 Seventh Avenue
New York, NY 10001
212-647-1890
www.aabt.org

The CFIDS Association of America (for those with chronic fatigue and immune dysfunction syndrome)
P.O. Box 220398
Charlotte, NC 28222-0398
704-365-2343
www.cfids.org

Children and Adults with Attention Deficit/Hyperactivity Disorder (CHADD)
8181 Professional Place, Suite 150
Landover, MD 20785
301-306-7070
National Resource Center on AD/HD: 800-233-4050
www.chadd.org

Crohn's & Colitis Foundation of America
386 Park Avenue South, 17th Floor
New York, NY 10016
800-932-2423
www.ccfa.org
info@ccfa.org

Depression and Bipolar Support Alliance
703 N. Franklin Street, Suite 501
Chicago, IL 60654-7225
800-826-3632
www.ndmda.org

Endometriosis Association
8585 N. 76th Place
Milwaukee, WI 53223
414-355-2200
www.endometriosisassn.org

Family Caregiver Alliance
180 Montgomery Street, Suite 1100
San Francisco, CA 94104
415-434-3388
800-445-8106
www.caregiver.org
info@caregiver.org

The Headache Society
19 Mantua Road
Mount Royal, NJ 08061
856-423-0043
www.americanheadachesociety.org
ahshq@talley.com

International Association for Women's Mental Health
8213 Lakenheath Way
Potomac, MD 20854
301-983-6282
iawmh@aol.com
www.iawmh.org

International Foundation for Functional Gastrointestinal Disorders
P.O. Box 170864
Milwaukee, WI 53217-8076
414-964-1799
888-964-2001
www.iffgd.org
iffgd@iffgd.org

Interstitial Cystitis Association
110 North Washington Street, Suite 340
Rockville, MD 20850
800-HELP-ICA (435-7422)
www.ichelp.org
ICAmail@ichelp.org

Mental Health America (formerly the National Mental Health Association)
2000 N. Beauregard Street, 6th Floor
Alexandria, VA 22311
703-684-7722
800-969-6642
www.nmha.org

Mood and Anxiety Disorders Program at NIMH (National Institute of Mental Health)
National Institutes of Health (NIH)
9000 Rockville Pike
Bethesda, MD 20892
866-627-6464
http://intramural.nimh.nih.gov/mood

National Alliance on Mental Illness (NAMI)
Colonial Place Three
2107 Wilson Boulevard, Suite 300
Arlington, VA 22201-3042
703-524-7600
www.nami.org

National Center for Post-Traumatic Stress Disorder
U.S. Department of Veterans Affairs
PTSD Information Center
802-296-6300
www.ncptsd.va.gov/ncmain/information
ncptsd@va.gov

National Fibromyalgia Association
2121 S. Towne Centre Place, Suite 300
Anaheim, CA 92806
714-921-0150
www.fmaware.org

National Institute of Mental Health (NIMH)
Science Writing, Press and Dissemination Branch
6001 Executive Boulevard, Room 8184, MSC 9663
Bethesda, MD 20892-9663
301-443-4513
866-615-6464
301-443-8431 (TTY)
866-415-8051 (TTY toll-free)
www.nimh.nih.gov/health/publications/index.shtml
nimhinfo@nih.gov

National Sleep Foundation
1522 K Street, N.W., Suite 500
Washington, DC 20005
202-347-3471
www.sleepfoundation.org
nsf@sleepfoundation.org

National Women's Health Resource Center (NWHRC)
157 Broad Street, Suite 106
Red Bank, NJ 07701
877-986-9472
www.healthywomen.org

Obsessive Compulsive Foundation
P.O. Box 961029
Boston, MA 02196
617-973–5801
www.ocfoundation.org
info@ocfoundation.org

Obsessive Compulsive Information Center
Madison Institute of Medicine
7617 Mineral Point Road, Suite 300
Madison, WI 53717
608-827-2470
www.miminc.org/aboutocic.asp
mim@miminc.org

Sidran Institute
200 East Joppa Road, Suite 207
Baltimore, MD 21286-3107
410-825-8888
888-825-8249
www.sidran.org
info@sidran.org

Society for Women's Health Research
1025 Connecticut Ave., N.W., Suite 701
Washington, DC 20036
202-223-8224
info@womenshealthresearch.org

The TMJ Association (for those with temporomandibular joint and muscle disorders, or TMJDs)
P.O. Box 26770
Milwaukee, WI 53226-0770
262-432-0350
www.tmj.org
info@tmj.org

NOTES

Introduction: In Defense of Anxiety

1. Associated Press, "Pentagon Totals Rise for Stress Disorder," *The New York Times,* May 28, 2008.

PART 1: ANXIETY: A GIRL'S BEST FRIEND—OR FOE?

Chapter 1: Anxiety's New Normal

1. "Women and Depression: A New View," University of New South Wales, May 17, 2001, at www.unsw.edu.au/news/pad/articles/2001/may/womenanddepression.html, accessed October 14, 2008.
2. B. S. McEwen, "Protection and Damage from Acute and Chronic Stress: Allostasis and Allostatic Overload and Relevance to the Pathophysiology of Psychiatric Disorders," *Annals of the New York Academy of Sciences* 1032 (2004):1–7.
3. V. Paquette, J. Lévesque, B. Mensour, J.-M. Leroux, G. Beaudoin, P. Bourgouin, and M. Beauregard, " 'Change the Mind and You Change the Brain': Effects of Cognitive-Behavioral Therapy on the Neural Correlates of Spider Phobia," *NeuroImage* 18, no. 2 (February 2003):401–409.

Chapter 2: "Am I Just a Worrier, or Is There Something Wrong with Me?"

1. Stephen S. Hall, "The Anatomy of Fear," *The New York Times Magazine*, February 28, 1999.
2. Ibid. Dr. Hooley's findings were preliminary and as yet unpublished as of the *Times* story's publication in 1999; the authors' attempt to contact Dr. Hooley to confirm publication was unsuccessful.
3. *Quick Reference to the Diagnostic Criteria from DSM-IV* (Washington, D.C.: American Psychiatric Association, 1994).

Chapter 3: It's Not Just in Your Head—It's in Your Brain (and the Rest of Your Body, Too)

1. For a detailed and entertaining exploration of the research, visit www.cns.nyu.edu/ledoux, website of the Center for Neural Science at NYU (LeDoux's lab). Also see Joseph LeDoux, *Synaptic Self: How Our Brains Become Who We Are* (New York: Viking, 2002).
2. S. E. Taylor, L. C. Klein, B. P. Lewis, T. L. Gruenewald, R. A. R. Gurung, and J. A. Updegraff, "Biobehavioral Responses to Stress in Females: Tend-and-Befriend, Not Fight-or-Flight," *Psychological Review* 107, no. 3 (2000):411–429.
3. Ibid.
4. Adapted from J. LeDoux, *The Emotional Brain: The Mysterious Underpinnings of Emotional Life* (New York: Simon & Schuster, 1996).
5. Ibid.
6. L. Vitetta, B. Anton, F. Cortizo, and A. Salt, "Mind-Body Medicine: Stress and Its Impact on Overall Health and Longevity," *Annals of the New York Academy of Sciences* 1057 (2005):492–505.
7. Ibid.
8. Ibid.
9. E. S. Epel, E. H. Blackburn, J. Lin, F. S. Dhabhar, N. E. Adler, J. D. Morrow, R. M. Cawthon, "Accelerated Telomere Shortening In Response to Life Stress," *Proceedings of the National Academy of Sciences of the United States of America* 101, no. 49 (2004):17312; "Chronic Stress Can Steal Years From Caregivers' Lifetimes," as reported on September 20, 2007, at www.sciencedaily.com/releases/2007/09/070918115543.htm, accessed on October 23, 2007.
10. L. M. Soravia, M. Heinrichs, A. Aerni, C. Maroni, G. Schelling, et al., "Glucocorticoids Reduce Phobic Fear in Humans," *Proceedings of the National Academy of Sciences of the United States of America* 103, no. 14 (2006):5585–5590.
11. S. Het and O. T. Wolf, "Mood Changes in Response to Psychosocial Stress

in Healthy Young Women: Effects of Pretreatment with Cortisol," *Behavioral Neuroscience* 121, no. 1 (2007):11–20.

12. A. M. Jasnow, J. Schulkin, and D. W. Pfaff, "Estrogen Facilitates Fear Conditioning and Increases Corticotropin-Releasing Hormone mRNA Expression in the Central Amygdala in Female Mice," *Hormones and Behavior* 49, no. 2 (2006):197–205.
13. R. Pearson and M. B. Lewis, "Fear Recognition Across the Menstrual Cycle," *Hormones and Behavior,* 47, no. 3 (2005):267–271.
14. M. K. Shear, M. Cloitre, D. Pine, and J. Ross, Introduction to "Women and Anxiety Disorders: Implications for Diagnosis and Treatment," Symposium Monograph Supplement, September 2004, based on proceedings from the Anxiety Disorders Association of America (ADAA) conference, "Women and Anxiety Disorders: Setting a Research Agenda," November 19–21, 2003.
15. Ibid.
16. "Women and Depression: A New View," University of New South Wales, May 17, 2001, at www.unsw.edu.au/news/pad/media/2001/may/womenanddepression.html, accessed July 16, 2007.
17. "Women and Anxiety Disorders," ADAA Symposium Monograph Supplement, September 2004.
18. K. Dillon and D. Brooks, "Unusual Cleaning Behavior in the Luteal Phase," *Psychological Reports* 70, no. 1 (1992):35–39.
19. M. Cloitre, "Women and Anxiety Disorders—Trauma and PTSD," ADAA Symposium Monograph Supplement, 2004.
20. Ibid.
21. T. Perlstein, "Women and Anxiety Disorders—P(re)M(enstrual) D(ysphoric) D(isorder)," ADAA Symposium Monograph Supplement, September 2004.
22. D. R. Kim, L. Gyulai, E. W. Freeman, M. F. Morrison, C. Baldassano, and B. Dube, "Premenstrual Dysphoric Disorder and Psychiatric Comorbidity," *Archives of Women's Mental Health* 7, no. 1 (2004):37–47, as cited by Perlstein, "PMDD," ADAA Symposium Monograph, September 2004.
23. M. Altemus and K. Brogan, "Women and Anxiety Disorders—Pregnancy and Postpartum," ADAA Symposium Monograph Supplement, September 2004.
24. Ibid.
25. "Hormones and Anxiety," as posted on the website of the Anxiety Disorders Association of America, www.adaa.org/ADAA%20web%20fin/Women&Hormones.pdf, accessed September 25, 2007.
26. Altemus and Brogan, "Pregnancy and Postpartum," ADAA Symposium Monograph Supplement, September 2004.

27. Ibid.
28. J. Heron, T. G. O'Connor, J. Evans, J. Golding, and V. Glover, "The Course of Anxiety and Depression Through Pregnancy and the Postpartum in a Community Sample," *Journal of Affective Disorders* 80 (2004): 65–73, as cited in Altemus and Brogan, "Pregnancy and Postpartum," ADAA Symposium Monograph Supplement, September 2004.
29. S. Matthey, B. Barnett, P. Howie, and D. J. Kavanagh, "Diagnosing Postpartum Depression in Mothers and Fathers: Whatever Happened to Anxiety?," *Journal of Affective Disorders* 74, no. 2 (April 2003):139–147; A. Wenzel, E. N. Haugen, L. C. Jackson, and K. Robinson, "Prevalence of Generalized Anxiety at Eight Weeks Postpartum," *Archives of Women's Mental Health* 6, no. 1 (2003):43–49; M. Muzik, C. M. Klier, L. Rosenblum, A. Holzinger, W. Umek, and H. Katschnig, *Acta Psychiatrica Scandinavica,* 102, no. 1 (July 2003):71–73, as cited in Altemus and Brogan, "Pregnancy and Postpartum."
30. M. Altemus, L. S. Redwine, Y. M. Leong, C. A. Frye, S. W. Porges, and C. S. Carter, "Responses to Laboratory Psychosocial Stress in Postpartum Women," *Psychosomatic Medicine,* 63 (2001):814–821, as cited in Altemus and Brogan, "Pregnancy and Postpartum."
31. J. W. Smoller, M. H. Pollack, S. Wassertheil-Smoller, B. Barton, S. L. Hendrix, R. D. Jackson, T. Dicken, A. Oberman, and D. S. Sheps, "Prevalence and Correlates of Panic Attacks in Postmenopausal Women," *Archives of Internal Medicine* 163 (2003):2041–2050.
32. Ibid.
33. J. W. Smoller, M. H. Pollack, S. Wassertheil-Smoller, R. D. Jackson, A. Oberman, N. D. Wong, D. Sheps, "Panic Attacks and Risk of Incident Cardiovascular Events Among Postmenopausal Women in the Women's Health Initiative Observational Study," *Archives of General Psychiatry* 64, no. 10 (2007):1153–1160.

PART 2: THE RELATIONSHIPS

1. Iris Murdoch, *A Severed Head,* 1961, as cited in *The Columbia Dictionary of Quotations,* ed. Robert Andrews (New York: Columbia University Press, 1993).

Chapter 4: The Reflexive-Impulsive Relationship

1. Janet Raloff, "Light Impacts: Hue and Timing Determine Whether Rays Are Beneficial or Detrimental," in *Science News Online,* www.sciencenews .org/articles/20060527/bob9.asp, accessed January 30, 2008.

Chapter 5: The Pervasive-Adaptive Relationship

1. "Irritable Bowel Syndrome," University of Illinois at Urbana-Champaign, at www.mckinley.uiuc.edu/handouts/irritable%5Fbowel%5Fsyndrome/irritable%5Fbowel%5Fsyndrome.html, accessed April 21, 2008.
2. R. B. Lydiard and S. A. Falsetti, "Experience with Anxiety and Depression Treatment Studies: Implications for Designing Irritable Bowel Syndrome Clinical Trials," *American Journal of Medicine* 107, no. 5 (1999):65–73.
3. D. S. Kaplan, P. S. Masand, and S. Gupta, "The Relationship of Irritable Bowel Syndrome and Panic Disorder," *Annals of Clinical Psychiatry* 8 (1996):81–88.

PART 3: MAKING IT BETTER: THE ROSS PRESCRIPTION

Chapter 8: Manage Your Anxiety, Improve Your Health

1. V. Benea, D. Muresian, L. Manolache, E. Robu, and J. D. Diaconu, "Stress and Atopic Dermatitis," *Dermatology and Psychosomatics* 2 (2001):205–207.
2. R. DeVogli, T. Chandola, and M. G. Marmot, "Negative Aspects of Close Relationships and Heart Disease," *Archives of Internal Medicine* 167 (2007): 1951–1957, as reported in "Study: Bad Marriage Could Damage Heart," www.cnn.com/2007/HEALTH/conditions/10/08/bad.marriage.heart.ap/index.html, accessed October 10, 2007.
3. E. D. Eaker, L. M. Sullivan, M. Shannon-Hayes, et al., "Marital Status, Marital Strain, and Risk of Coronary Heart Disease or Total Mortality: The Framingham Offspring Study," *Psychosomatic Medicine* 69 (2007): 509–513, as reported in Tara Parker-Pope, "Well: Marital Spats, Taken to Heart," *The New York Times,* October 2, 2007.
4. E. S. Epel, E. H. Blackburn, J. Lin, F. S. Dhabhar, N. E. Adler, J. D. Morrow, and R. M. Cawthon, "Accelerated Telomere Shortening in Response to Life Stress," *Proceedings of the National Academy of Sciences of the United States of America* 101, no. 49 (2004):17312.
5. "Chronic Stress Can Steal Years from Caregivers' Lifetimes," as reported on September 20, 2007, at www.sciencedaily.com/releases/2007/09/070918115543.htm, accessed on October 23, 2007.
6. "Irritable Bowel Syndrome," University of Illinois at Urbana-Champaign, at www.mckinley.uiuc.edu/handouts/irritable_bowel_syndrome/irritable_bowel_syndrome.html, accessed on December 8, 2008.
7. S. C. Ganguli, M. C. Kamath, M. Mohammed, Y. Chen, E. J. Irvine, S. M. Collins, and G. Tougas, "Patients with Ulcerative Colitis (UC) Demonstrate Abnormalities of Autonomic Function Which Are Correlated with Measures of Anxiety," as reported in Louise Gagnon,

"Study Suggests Link Between Anxiety and Ulcerative Colitis Flare: Presented at C[anadian] D[igestive] D[iseases] W[eek]," www.docguide.com/news/content.nsf/news/8525697700573E1885256B56006F68B1?Open&id=48DDE4A73E09A969852568880078C249&count=10, accessed May 2, 2008.
8. David Kohn, "Psychotherapy for All: An Experiment," *The New York Times,* March 11, 2008.
9. Alex Berenson, "Drug Approved. Is Disease Real?", *The New York Times,* January 14, 2008.
10. Ibid.
11. Ibid.
12. C. M. Albert, C. U. Chae, K. M. Rexrode, J. E. Manson, and I. Kawachi, "Phobic Anxiety and Risk of Coronary Heart Disease and Sudden Cardiac Death Among Women," *Circulation* 111 (2005):480–487.
13. Marianne Legato, *Eve's Rib* (New York: Harmony Books, 2002).
14. R. D. Goodwin, F. Jacobi, and W. Thefeld, "Mental Disorders and Asthma in the Community," *Archives of General Psychiatry* 60 (2003):1125–1130.
15. According to a 2007 joint study by researchers at the University of Washington School of Medicine and Seattle Children's Hospital Research Institute, cited in "Asthma Linked to Anxiety and Depressive Disorders, Study Suggests," *Science Daily,* November 7, 2007, at www.healthyplace.com/communities/anxiety/news_2007/asthma.asp, accessed April 16, 2008.
16. O. Palesh, L. D. Butler, C. Koopman, J. Giese-Davis, R. Carlson, and D. Spiegel, "Stress History and Breast Cancer Recurrence," *Journal of Psychosomatic Research* 63, no. 3 (September 2007):233–239.
17. P. P. Roy-Byrne, K. W. Davidson, R. C. Kessler, G. J. G. Asmundson, R. D. Goodwin, L. Kubzansky, R. B. Lydiard, M. J. Massie, W. Katon, S. K. Laden, and M. B. Stein, "Anxiety Disorders and Comorbid Medical Illness," *General Hospital Psychiatry* Volume 30, Issue 3, May–June 2008, 208–225.
18. Ibid.
19. C. M. Bulik, P. F. Sullivan, F. A. Carter, and P. R. Joyce, "Lifetime Anxiety Disorders in Women with Bulimia Nervosa," *Comprehensive Psychiatry* 37, no. 5 (1996):368–374; C. Thornton and J. Russell, "Obsessive-Compulsive Comorbidity in the Dieting Disorders," *International Journal of Eating Disorders* 21, no. 1 (1997):83–87; M. A. Tsivil'ko, M. V. Korkina, A. E. Briukhin, S. D. Bushenina, and T. Lineva, "Obsessive-Phobic Disorders in Anorexia and Bulimia Nervosa," *Zh Nevropatol Psikhiatr Im S S Korsakova* 97, no. 3 (1997):16–19, as cited in "Eating Disorders and Anxiety Disorders," http://panicdisorder.about.com/cs/comorbiddisorders/a/eatingdisorders.htm, accessed May 22, 2008.
20. W. H. Kaye, C. M. Bulik, L. Thornton, N. Barbarich, K. Masters, and the

Price Foundation Collaborative Group, "Comorbidity of Anxiety Disorders with Anorexia and Bulimia Nervosa," *The American Journal of Psychiatry* 161 (December 2004):2215–2221.

21. Kimberly Pulse, "The Comorbidity of Anxiety Disorders and Eating Disorders," at www.vanderbilt.edu/AnS/psychology/health_psychology/AnxietyandEatingDisorders.html, accessed May 21, 2008.
22. Statistics cited by the South Carolina Department of Mental Health, "Eating Disorder Statistics," at www.state.sc.us/dmh/anorexia/statistics.htm, accessed May 23, 2008.
23. E. S. Becker, J. Margraf, V. Turke, U. Soeder, and S. Neumer, "Obesity and Mental Illness in a Representative Sample of Young Women," *International Journal of Obesity* 25, suppl. 1 (May 2001):S5–S9.
24. S. E. Anderson, P. Cohen, E. N. Naumova, and A. Must, "Association of Depression and Anxiety Disorders with Weight Change in a Prospective Community-Based Study of Children Followed Up into Adulthood," *Archives of Pediatrics and Adolescent Medicine* 160 (2006):285–291, as cited in "Depression, Anxiety in Girls Linked to Higher Body Mass Index in Women" at www.emaxhealth.com/25/4733.html, accessed May 23, 2008.
25. "Substance Use and Mood and Anxiety Disorders Among the Most Prevalent Psychiatric Disorders," at www.medicalnewstoday.com/articles/11578.php, accessed May 28, 2008.
26. "Anxiety and Illicit Drug Use Link Found," reprinted from www.psychiatrymatters.md.

Chapter 10: The Ross Prescription, Part 2: Taking Action

1. E. D. Eaker, L. M. Sullivan, M. Shannon-Hayes, et al., "Marital Status, Marital Strain, and Risk of Coronary Heart Disease or Total Mortality: The Framingham Offspring Study," *Psychosomatic Medicine* 69 (2007): 509–513, as reported in Tara Parker-Pope, "Well: Marital Spats, Taken to Heart," *The New York Times,* October 2, 2007.
2. R. H. Cox, T. R. Thomas, P. S. Hinton, and O. M. Donahue, "Effects of Acute 60 and 80% VO_2 Max Bouts of Aerobic Exercise on State of Anxiety of Women of Different Age Groups Across Time," *Research Quarterly for Exercise and Sport* 75, no. 2 (June 2004):165–175, as cited in "High-Intensity Exercise Best for Anxiety," WebMD Health News, www.webmd.com/anxiety-panic/news/20030716/high-intensity-exercise-best-for-anxiety, accessed June 11, 2008.
3. G. Simon, M. VonKorff, and W. Barlow, "Health Care Costs of Primary Care Patients with Recognized Depression," *Archives of General Psychiatry,* 52 (1995):850–852.

4. A. Ströhle, C. Feller, M. Onken, F. Godemann, A. Heinz, and F. Dimeo, "The Acute Antipanic Activity of Aerobic Exercise," *The American Journal of Psychiatry* 162, no. 12 (2005):2376–2378.
5. For more, see "Depression and Anxiety: Exercise Eases Symptoms" at www.mayoclinic.com/health/depression-and-exercise/MH00043, accessed June 12, 2008.

FURTHER READING

These volumes were a valuable resource in the writing of this book:

Brizendine, Louann. *The Female Brain.* New York: Morgan Road Books, 2006.
DeRosis, Helen A. *Women and Anxiety.* New York: Hatherleigh Press, 1998.
Kornstein, Susan G., and Anita H. Clayton. *Women's Mental Health.* New York: The Guilford Press, 2002.
LeDoux, Joseph. *The Emotional Brain.* New York: Simon & Schuster Paperbacks, 1996.
———. *Synaptic Self.* New York: Viking, 2002.
Legato, Marianne J. *Eve's Rib.* New York: Harmony Books, 2002.
Lerner, Harriet. *The Dance of Fear.* New York: Perennial Currents, 2005.
Ross, Jerilyn. *Triumph Over Fear.* New York: Bantam Books, 1994.

INDEX

ABOUT THE AUTHORS

Jerilyn Ross, M.A., is one of the nation's leading experts on anxiety disorders. An active psychotherapist, patient advocate, and author, she is director of the Ross Center for Anxiety & Related Disorders in Washington, D.C., and president and CEO of the Anxiety Disorders Association of America.

Ross received her graduate training in psychology from the New School for Social Research in New York City and began her clinical practice and public advocacy activities in 1978. Since then she has appeared on more than three hundred television and radio shows, including *Nightline, Dateline, Anderson Cooper 360, 20/20, Today, Good Morning America, The Oprah Winfrey Show, Larry King Live,* and *The Diane Rehm Show.* From 1987 to 1992, she hosted an award-winning weekly talk show on WRC radio in Washington, D.C.

A member of the American Psychological Association and the Association for Behavioral and Cognitive Therapies, Ross frequently conducts public and professional lectures, seminars, and workshops on anxiety disorders. She has been the subject of feature profiles in *The Washington Post Magazine, Biography Magazine,* and *The Economics of Neuroscience* (*TEN*) and is frequently quoted in *The New York Times, The Wall Street Journal, The Boston Globe, The Washington Post, Chicago Sun-Times,* and *Chicago Tribune.* She has contributed to *The American Journal of Psychiatry* and *The Journal of Clinical Psychiatry* as well as several books, and has been interviewed by numerous popular magazines, including *Time, Newsweek, U.S. News & World Report, BusinessWeek, Vogue, Glamour, Self, Harper's Bazaar, Reader's Digest, Ladies' Home Journal, Good Housekeeping,* and *Parade.* She also developed a comprehensive audio-video self-help program, *Freedom from Anxiety,* and is the author of *Triumph Over Fear: A Book of Help and Hope for People with Anxiety, Panic Attacks, and Phobias.*

As ADAA president, Ross has twice testified before Congress on behalf of the millions of Americans who suffer from an anxiety disorder, and has served on several advisory committees for the National Institute of Mental Health.

Ross has received many honors, including the 2004 Patient Advocacy Award from the American Psychiatric Association, the 2001 Anxiety Disorder Initiative Award from the World Council on Anxiety and the World Psychiatric Association, a 2000 Telly Award, and a 1994 Distinguished Humanitarian Award from the American Association of Applied and Preventive Psychology.

Ross lives in Potomac, Maryland, with her husband, Ron Cohen.

ROBIN CANTOR-COOKE is the co-author of *Satisfaction* (with Anita H. Clayton, M.D.) and *Thriving with Heart Disease* (with Wayne M. Sotile, Ph.D.) and the ghostwriter of a *New York Times* number one bestseller. She has worked as a writer, editor, scriptwriter, and producer on more than forty books and tape programs and is an adjunct faculty member at the College of William & Mary. She lives with her husband and two sons in Williamsburg, Virginia.